Counselling and Psychology
for Health Professionals

THERAPY IN PRACTICE SERIES

Edited by Jo Campling

This series of books is aimed at 'therapists' concerned with rehabilitation in a very broad sense. The intended audience particularly includes occupational therapists, physiotherapists and speech therapists, but many titles will also be of interest to nurses, psychologists, medical staff, social workers, teachers or volunteer workers. Some volumes are interdisciplinary, others are aimed at one particular profession. All titles will be comprehensive but concise and practical but with due reference to relevant theory and evidence. They are not research monographs but focus on professional practice, and will be of value to both students and qualified personnel.

Counselling and Psychology for Health Professionals

Edited by

Rowan Bayne

Lecturer in Psychology and Counselling,
University of East London, UK

and

Paula Nicolson

Lecturer in Medical Psychology,
Sheffield University, UK

CHAPMAN & HALL

London · Glasgow · New York · Tokyo · Melbourne · Madras

Published by Chapman & Hall, 2-6 Boundary Row, London SE1 8HN

Chapman & Hall, 2-6 Boundary Row, London SE1 8HN, UK

Blackie Academic & Professional, Wester Cleddens Road, Bishopbriggs, Glasgow G64 2NZ, UK

Chapman & Hall, 29 West 35th Street, New York NY10001, USA

Chapman & Hall Japan, Thomson Publishing Japan, Hirakawacho Nemoto Building, 6F, 1-7-11 Hirakawa-cho, Chiyoda-ku, Tokyo 102, Japan

Chapman & Hall Australia, Thomas Nelson Australia, 102 Dodds Street, South Melbourne, Victoria 3205, Australia

Chapman & Hall India, R. Seshadri, 32 Second Main Road, CIT East, Madras 600 035, India

Distributed in the USA and Canada by Singular Publishing Group Inc., 4284 41st Street, San Diego, California 92105

First edition 1993

©1993 Chapman & Hall

Typeset in 10/12pt Palatino by ROM Data Corporation Ltd. Cornwall
Printed in Great Britain by Page Bros, Norwich

ISBN 0 412 41140 7   1 56593 117 3 (USA)

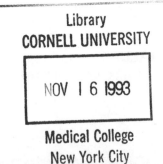

For Philip Greenway
and
Derry Nicolson

Contents

Contributors

Dr Michael Barkham
Research Clinical Psychologist
MRC/ESRC Applied and Social Psychology Unit
Sheffield University

Dr Rowan Bayne
Lecturer in Psychology and Counselling
Psychology Department
University of East London

Jenny Bimrose
Head of the Centre for Training in Careers Guidance
Psychology Department
University of East London

Tim Bond
Staff Tutor in Counselling
Department of Adult and Continuing Education
University of Durham

Dr Julian Boon
Forensic Psychologist
Department of Psychology
Leicester University

Dr Jan Burns
Lecturer in Clinical Psychology
and Principal Clinical Psychologist,
Bradford District Health Authority
Department of Psychiatry
University of Leeds

Professor Graham Davies
Head of the Department of Psychology
Leicester University

Dr Stephen Frosh
Senior Lecturer in Psychology
Department of Psychology
London University

Ian Horton
Senior Lecturer in Counselling and Psychotherapy
Psychology Department
University of East London

Chris Lewis
Principal Lecturer in Occupational Psychology
Psychology Department
University of East London

Dr Harriette Marshall
Senior Lecturer in Social Psychology
Psychology Department
University of East London

Dr Paula Nicolson
Lecturer in Medical Psychology
Department of Psychiatry
University of Sheffield

Elizabeth Noon
Research Associate
Department of Psychology
Leicester University

Dr Keith Phillips
Head of the Department of Psychology
University of East London

Dr Jonathan Smith
Lecturer in Psychology
Department of Psychology
Keele University

Dr Jane Ussher
Lecturer in Psychology
Psychology Division
School of Cultural and Community Studies
University of Sussex

Dr David White
Principal Lecturer in Developmental Psychology
Psychology Department
University of East London

Dr Anne Woollett
Deputy Head of the Department of Psychology
University of East London

Acknowledgements

We would like to thank the following people for their contributions to the development of this book or particular chapters : Susamma Ajith, Jo Campling, Terri Cooper, Geoffrey Dean, Ian Horton, Jean Kummerow and Lynne Mallinson.

Table 3.4 first appeared in the *Bulletin of Psychological Type*.

Rowan Bayne and Paula Nicolson

Introduction

This book is for trainee and experienced health professionals. It outlines and discusses practical skills, ideas and evidence from counselling and psychology, and is intended to help practitioners increase their effectiveness, confidence and well-being. In this introduction we would like to say something about three things: why we chose the topics we did, how we see the book being useful, and the book's structure.

CHOICE OF TOPICS

We chose topics that met several criteria. First, health professionals on our courses wanted to know about them in more depth than a basic textbook can provide. Second, we knew someone who was an expert, would write clearly about them, and would (probably) meet deadlines. Third, they were not readily available in a concise, practical, up to date form.

Many valuable topics were ruled out by this third criterion, e.g. coping with stress (Bond, 1986; Fontana, 1989), coping with loss (Parry, 1990), counselling patients with different illnesses (Davis and Fallowfield, 1991), basic counselling skills (Burnard, 1989; Nicolson and Bayne, 1990), assertiveness (Dickson, 1987), detailed case histories (Yalom, 1989), particular orientations to counselling (Dryden, 1990; Mearns and Thorne, 1988), and so on.

USING THIS BOOK

This book, then, is intended to complement basic and other texts. Its particular value lies in its emphasis on application, the unusual nature of some of its topics and its expert, concise summaries of more orthodox ones.

It is not, therefore, a book which you need necessarily read straight through. Rather, we think health professionals will choose to 'dip into it' on various levels and on many occasions: studying for exams, writing essays, and most often to support practice.

It provides:

1. skills, strategies and frameworks, e.g. before a counselling supervision session (Chapter 2); to help prevent violence (4); to clarify a view about the role of social context, and to put that view itself in context (10);
2. ideas or evidence that might be useful to a client or oneself, e.g. a baffled step-parent (Chapter 8); someone struggling with stereotypes about being 'middle-aged' or 'old' (12); someone (client, manager, self) who asks: 'What is counselling? Is it any good? Is it cost-effective?' (5).

STRUCTURE OF THE BOOK

One of the most enjoyable but frustrating aspects of editing the book was trying out different structures and sequences.

Each was compelling and obvious for a while – until one of us saw a flaw or a way that seemed better. The present structure is also flawed : using research (Chapter 14) and social context (Chapter 9), for example, could well be in the section on counselling practice, but both also serve a 'setting in context' function in their respective sections. Sections and chapters are as follows:

Section One : Counselling Practice

This section begins with Tim Bond's analysis of counselling and counselling skills. He argues that the overall effect of making this distinction can be a liberating one, leading to clearer communications and less role conflict and confusion. Second, Ian Horton takes a very positive view of counselling supervision, seeing it as an opportunity for practitioners to develop their *own* styles of counselling (rather than a method of inspection and control). He outlines in detail several strategies for supervisees to choose from. Third, Rowan Bayne suggests applications of a theory of personality to both informal and professional conversations, and to understanding oneself and others more clearly and constructively. Fourth, Jan Burns discusses potential violence, at work and on home visits, offering practical advice on preventing it, and on coping if prevention fails. Fifth, Michael Barkham reviews the research on the effectiveness of counselling, and then provides practical guidelines for practitioners who wish to evaluate their own counselling and to make out a case for more resources.

Section Two : Families

The second section contains four chapters. Anne Woollett discusses research and ideas on becoming a parent, pregnancy and infertility. David White analyses some of the effects of divorce on adults and children and, in the following chapter, what is known about the 'reconstituted' and 'blended' families which often result, and the implications for stepmothers, stepfathers and those who work professionally with them. Stephen Frosh reviews current information on child sexual abusers and victims, factors for practitioners to take into account, and interventions.

Section Three : Social Context

In the opening chapter for this section, Jenny Bimrose proposes a framework which acknowledges several perspectives on the role of social context in counselling. The framework enables practitioners to locate and consider their own positions on this issue, one which psychology and counselling has tended to neglect. The other four chapters in this section provide further examples of the relevance of social context to understanding behaviour and to effective interventions. First, Jane Ussher summarizes the various approaches to psychopathology and then criticizes them as ignoring both social context and individual experience. Second, Paula Nicolson challenges stereotypes about women and men from midlife to old age, and draws out some of their implications for practitioners. Third, Keith Phillips reviews attempts to prevent AIDS with large-scale health education campaigns, and argues instead for local, targeted approaches with particular groups, taking each group's sexual needs, practices and pleasures into account. There is a major role for health prefessionals here in devising, communicating and evaluating such campaigns. Fourth, Julian Boon, Graham Davies and Elizabeth Noon clarify the legal status of children in court – a barrier to working effectively with them – and suggest strategies, based on extensive research, for helping children cope in this unusual context.

Section Four : Research and Practitioners

We want this section to demystify research and to encourage more health professionals to take it seriously in their practice and also to do it. In the opening chapter, Chris Lewis argues that everyone does research (what differs is the degree of formality and rigour) and suggests ways of making sense of papers and articles on psychology and counselling. Harriette Marshall uses research on maternity care to illustrate the view that discourse analysis has advantages over standard questionnaires for understanding attitudes. Jonathan Smith reviews the case study in research and practice. All three authors see health professionals as being in an excellent position to carry out research which is valuable for themselves, their clients and their colleagues.

REFERENCES

Bond, M. (1986) *Stress and Self-awareness : A guide for nurses*, Heinemann, London.

Burnard, P. (1989) *Counselling Skills for Health Professionals*, Chapman and Hall, London.

Davis, H. and Fallowfield, L. (1991) (eds.) *Counselling and Communication in Health Care*, Wiley, Chichester.

Dickson, A. (1987) *A Woman in Your Own Right: Assertiveness and you*, Quartet, London.

Dryden, W. (ed.) (1990) *Individual Therapy: A handbook*, Open University Press, Milton Keynes.

Fontana, D. (1989) *Managing Stress*, BPS/Routledge, London.

Mearns, D. and Thorne, B. (1988) *Person-Centred Counselling in Action*, Sage, London.

Nicolson, P. and Bayne, R. (1990) *Applied Psychology for Social Workers*, 2nd edn, Macmillan, London.

Parry, G. (1990) *Coping with Crises*, BPS/Routledge, London.

Yalom, I.D. (1989) *Love's Executioner and Other Tales of Psychotherapy*, Penguin, London.

Section One

Counselling Practice

Counselling, counselling skills and professional roles

Tim Bond

Any exploration of the relationship between counselling, counselling skills and professional roles raises fundamental questions about the nature of counselling. For instance, when an occupational therapist offers counselling to a patient, what should that patient expect? How would the counselling being offered be different from a doctor advising a patient how to improve her health or a nurse listening to a patient's worries about being away from home, or a medical social worker helping with problems about the patient returning home? Is counselling something which should only be offered by someone with the occupational title of 'counsellor' or can the role be undertaken by people with other professional roles? This chapter argues that the answers to these questions are becoming clearer and that it is now possible to map the relationship between counselling, counselling skills and professional roles.

MEANING OF THE TERM 'COUNSELLING'

There is no copyright or patent on the use of the term 'counselling'. In the wider community the term 'counselling' is often used to mean advice-giving, typically the expert advice of a professional. The Concise Oxford Dictionary (Sykes, 1987) still defines counselling in this way. It is therefore not surprising to find that amongst the caring professions, particularly medicine, there is still a view of counselling as the current popular term for giving advice to people. However, a recent report on HIV counselling cited evidence that this view is declining and that the term 'counselling' is increasingly being used to describe a less directive way of helping people which can usefully be distinguished from other forms of help (Bond, 1991). A comparison between a historical definition deduced by academic analysis in the USA and a recent definition used within the largest organization of counsellors in Britain assists in drawing out some of the main elements of a current British understanding of the term 'counselling'.

During the height of the Californian personal growth movement when the term 'counselling' was gaining popular usage in therapeutic psychology, Gustad (1953) reviewed historical definitions of counselling and identified three main categories: the participants were usually relating one to one, the counsellor having some professional role, e.g. health worker, teacher, minister, psychologist; the goals of counselling were described in terms of improved adjustment or higher functioning; and the definitions stressed learning outcomes, such as improved social skills. With these ingredients he produced the following definition:

> 'Counselling is a learning-oriented process, carried on in a simple, one-to-one social environment, in which a counsellor, professionally competent and with relevant psychological skills and knowledge, seeks to assist a client by methods appropriate to the latter's needs ... to learn more about himself, to learn how to put such understanding into effect in relation to more clearly perceived, realistically defined goals to the end that the client may become a happier and more productive member of his society.'
>
> (Gustad, 1953)

This definition compares with the latest definition of counselling used by the British Association for Counselling (BAC):

> 'Counselling is a skilled and principled use of relationships which develops self-knowledge, emotional acceptance and growth and personal resources. The overall aim is to live more fully and satisfyingly. Counselling may be concerned with addressing and resolving specific problems, making decisions, coping with crises, working through feelings and inner conflict, or improving relationships with others.

The counsellor's role is to facilitate the client's work in ways that respect the client's values, personal resources, and capacity for self-determination.'

(British Association for Counselling, 1990).

Despite the development of these two definitions in different cultures and times, they have much in common. In both, 'counselling' is defined in terms of what counsellors do and what is done is described in terms of goals and learning outcomes. Both contain the broader aim of improved human effectiveness expressed respectively as 'becoming a happier and more productive member of his society', and 'to live more fully and satisfyingly.' The achievement of this broader aim by the client requires both a learning of expertise in a particular cultural context and a sense of purpose in the application of that expertise.

Such a sense of purpose was labelled 'intentionality' by Ivey and Simek-Downing (1980) in their analysis of the goals of counselling. The label raises a fundamental question: whose sense of purpose or intentionality is being implemented in counselling – the counsellor's or the client's? The answer is implicit in Gustad's definition. However, the answer is so important in the British context that Gustad's 'appropriate' is elaborated into facilitating 'in ways that respect the client's values, personal resources and capacity for self-determination', and is made more visible by dividing the definition into paragraphs.

Recent research into counselling in a variety of settings provides some insight into why respect for the client's values, personal resources and capacity for self-determination has become so prominent in the British experience of counselling. The research shows that this touchstone of counselling is not yet well understood by non-counsellors and even by some counsellors. This lack of understanding is a source of frustration for many counsellors, and therefore increases the importance they attach to communicating their methodology more effectively.

RESPECT FOR THE CLIENT'S CAPACITY FOR SELF-DETERMINATION

A recent study of cancer counsellors from a variety of settings, including hospital, hospice, community and voluntary organizations, showed that the goal of empowering their clients could not be established without extensive training. Roberts and Fallowfield found that the self-expressed goals of 219 counsellors could be grouped into three main categories according to whether they were orientated to: (a) service provision, (b) empowering the client, or (c) having patients/clients respond as staff wish. They found an association between the expression of goals orientated towards empowering the client and whether the counsellor held recognised psychotherapy or counselling qualifications, e.g. diplomas, certificates or degrees in counselling, clinical psychology, psychiatry, nursing with RMN qualifications and social work. However, there was no relationship between the respondents' stated goals and whether they had merely attended a counselling course of any description, particularly short courses.

The authors commented, 'This in itself is not surprising. Many of the courses which our respondents were prepared to recommend were very short and could not by themselves be expected to produce lasting change in attitude or practice' (Roberts and Fallowfield, 1990). A corollary to their findings is that empowering the client in ways which respect their capacity for self-determination is not a usual goal for staff working with cancer patients unless they have a significant commitment to and training in counselling. It would seem that, all too often, patients are expected to conform to institutional procedures or shape their emotional responses to a previously determined template reiterated by undertrained counsellors.

The same issue emerged in a different way in a study of HIV counsellors (Bond, 1991). As part of an initiative to promote good practice in this newly developing area of work, the AIDS Unit of the Department of Health sponsored a joint project with BAC which involved consultations with 142 HIV counsellors from the health service, social services, voluntary organisations and a variety of other agencies. During the formal consultation procedure a majority of HIV counsellors reported frustration that their commitment to working in ways which respect their clients' capacity for self-determination was not more widely understood by colleagues. Failure to appreciate the client-orientated nature of their work meant that counsellors often felt subjected to inappropriate expectations. In particular, they expressed unease at being expected to obtain the client's compliance with social or institutional policies regardless of the client's wishes. The most widely reported cause of role conflict for HIV counsellors arose from their participation in HIV prevention programmes. Fortunately, most clients are concerned to protect themselves and others from HIV infection.

In these circumstances there is no conflict between the counsellor's objectives and the client's self-determination objectives. However, a minority of clients appear unconcerned about minimizing the transmission of HIV which caused the counsellors considerable role conflict. In these circumstances the counsellor has a choice between two unsatisfactory options: either continuing to respect the client's capacity for self-determination, and thus creating an ethical conflict for the counsellor with the values of the wider community; or else becoming more confrontational and risking both the destruction of their relationship with the client and compromising the values of counselling. The HIV counsellors feared their difficulty in working with a minority of clients could discredit their client-orientated way of working which is so important to intervening effectively with the majority of clients. Respect for the client's values, personal resources and capacity for self-determination are the cornerstones of establishing trusting and effective relationships with most client groups, but particularly with people concerned about HIV, because of their extreme vulnerability to social rejection (Bond, 1991).

The potential for role conflict is not confined to counsellors working in health settings. There is a similar potential for role conflict in educational settings. In a study conducted in a British university by Pashley (1976), he found different expectations of the student counselling services depending on whether they were being considered from a staff or student viewpoint. Lecturers and administrators wanted the service to be an adjunct to the psychiatric services, providing a minority of students with a form of crisis intervention without which academic or emotional breakdown might occur. They did not want what the students wanted: an independent, neutral counselling service which was operated to change organizational structures as well as individual coping strategies, which was closer to the role that the counsellors would have chosen for themselves. In a more recent survey of counselling in further and higher education in the UK, Glynis Breakwell found that the student counsellors were aware of this disparity between the objectives of the students and the institution:

'The emphasis for the individual is upon providing academic and emotional support and engendering personal growth and self-exploration. For the institution the focus is improving academic performance (manifested in reduced student failure rates) and improving the institutional ambience (a healthier learning environment).'

(Breakwell, 1987).

In different ways, each of these studies demonstrates that counsellors attach considerable importance to working in ways which respect and enhance the client's capacity for self-determination. It is also evident that this central tenet of counselling is not always convenient and can create the potential for conflict between the clients' objectives and those of colleagues and the institution.

A corollary of working in ways which respect the clients' capacity for self-determination is the emphasis counsellors place on acknowledging the clients' power within the counselling relationship by entering into clearly negotiated contracts about confidentiality, the duration of the relationship and other terms on which counselling is offered (BAC, 1990). The explicit nature of the agreement between the counsellor and client was central to an earlier definition of counselling that served quite a different function.

'People become engaged in counselling when a person, occupying regularly or temporarily the role of counsellor, offers or agrees explicitly to offer time, attention and respect to another person or persons temporarily in the role of client,'

(BAC, 1985)

At that time the focus on the term 'explicitly' was considered important as the 'dividing line between the counselling task and "ad hoc" counselling and is the major safeguard of the rights of the consumer' (BAC, 1985). In more recent years this distinction between formal counselling and ad hoc counselling has been renamed and become the boundary marker between counselling and the use of counselling skills.

THE USE OF COUNSELLING SKILLS

As the term 'counselling' has become increasingly more specific, and therefore more exclusive, a need has arisen to find a way of labelling the role many professionals and volunteers take on when they are applying the methods and values of counselling to working with people in relationships other than that of counsellor and client, e.g. nurse-patient, psychologist-client, tutor-student, doctor-patient, etc. An increasingly accepted term for this role is 'using counselling skills'. This has been formally recognized within the British Association for Counselling by the production of a Code of Ethics and Practice for Counselling Skills (BAC, 1989) which is more flexible and less specific than the Code for Counsellors (BAC, 1990). The process of preparing the ground for a code for counselling skills involved a debate which paralleled the insights into skills developed within psychology (Argyle, 1981).

A naive approach to identifying counselling skills is to list all the skills borrowed from counselling. However this approach is quickly frustrated because the list looks indistinguishable from any other list of communication skills used in any other professional caring role. In response to an article (Bond, 1989) attempting to define counselling skills, John Pratt succinctly made the point that what distinguishes different kinds of skills is the objective of the user: 'Skills ... cannot, by definition, be value-free. They are the means by which people with particular sets of values achieve their objects'.

These values, integral to the use of counselling skills, present a considerable challenge to the helper. John Pratt questioned:

'Whose power and autonomy, whose 'brainwork' and perspective of the adverse situation discussed does the helping process primarily gauge? Most professional helping is about advising or informing if not actually treating or handling a person's body. Counselling attempts to re-affirm the individual's experience of and control over his own life. In many basic counselling courses I have taught this is the most difficult thing for nurses and most other health carers to simulate and act on. It is significant for them when they understand this and begin to feel free *not* to search desperately in their own minds for an "answer" to their client's problems but concentrate instead on "staying with" their client's experience. In using counselling skills as part of their work, professional helpers have consciously to move between these and other modes of helping.'

(Pratt, 1990)

Therefore the user of counselling skills shares with the counsellor the potential for role conflict arising from similar causes. However, users of counselling skills may experience a more acute sense of role conflict arising from the values intrinsic in counselling skills and those of their main role, as the boundaries which usually define a counselling relationship are unlikely to be present. For instance, in the use of counselling skills, there are usually no standardized ways for making an offer of time and availability, managing the time, negotiating the terms on which help is being offered particularly with regard to confidentiality which may be compromised by the plurality of roles, and the importance of independent supervision and support. Even though these boundary markers are usually absent during the use of counselling skills, it cannot be assumed that they are always present during counselling. An optimum level of counselling practice is not yet universally implemented, although there is increasing agreement about what these standards should be. The creation of the concept of counselling skills has had a two-pronged effect. Firstly, it has drawn attention to the importance of valuing the client's capacity for self-determination when using counselling skills and revived interest in the relevance of these values to other forms of helping. Secondly, the distinction between counselling skills and counselling has created the conceptual space for a more specific use of the term 'counselling'.

COUNSELLING AND PROFESSIONAL ROLES

The meaning of counselling has narrowed to the specific activity or role which may be undertaken only when there is an explicit contract to work with the methods and values consistent with counselling. As the definition of counselling has narrowed, it is no longer possible to think of counselling as everything performed by someone with the occupational role of counsellor. The role of counsellor is typically a subrole within a broader occupational role, which in both the USA and UK may include a considerable number of different professions, e.g. psychiatric nurse, occupational therapist, clinical psychologist, minister, tutor, etc. All these occupational roles provide a useful background in different ways of helping people including counselling. However, there is also potential for confusion between roles. Therefore the practitioner requires acute awareness of the shifts in role and an ability to communicate these changes. Clear communication both to clients and to colleagues helps to minimize role conflict and confusion of expectations about the service being offered. Even when someone is employed as a counsellor, it is unlikely that all their time is spent working with clients in ways compatible with counselling. Typically, counsellors are also engaged in training, research and administration as well as other subroles.

As the meaning of the term 'counselling' has become more specialized, the opportunity for professionalization of the role has increased. Inevitably there are mixed feelings about this trend. Some people fear that this will involve distancing counselling from clients and creating a mystique of expertise which could be incompatible with the fundamental values of counselling, particularly respect for the client's integrity. Others fear that in formalizing the helping process, something which is an everyday human function has been ritualized into unnecessarily elaborate specialities. On the other hand there is growing recognition that any serious attempt to ensure adequate competence and accountability of counsellors involves some professionalization.

Belonging to different occupational groups, counsellors address these issues in ways which vary between occupations. The broad transoccupational considerations will most probably continue to be discussed within the forum of the British Association for Counselling. However, some occupations may work in advance of this forum, and in doing so may gain some advantage in credibility and capacity to secure employment in counselling. Counselling psychologists, who have charter status within the British Psychological Society (BPS), have this advantage. The process of achieving charter status has involved creating an infrastructure of procedures to establish standards of training, complaints procedures, etc. to ensure accountability and competence. There also appears to be an internal dynamic within the BPS which ensures that each specialism within psychology, including counselling psychology, lives up to the standards of the others.

Within the 'broader church' of the British Association for Counselling, which includes many occupational groups and voluntary counsellors, the process of addressing issues about achieving accountability and competence is inevitably more protracted. However, the participation of counselling psychologists at this forum adds to the rich experience of counsellors with other professional backgrounds. The evidence of the various surveys of the state of counselling in different settings referred to earlier in this chapter suggests that issues about training and supervision remain extremely important to establishing the credibility of the counselling role.

The training of counsellors has developed into an issue in national and potentially European social policy. In 1991, the Department of Employment started a mapping exercise with a view to establishing some national standards for the basic training in counselling skills within professional training. It is anticipated that once this exercise is completed, attention may turn towards counselling training. At the same time, there are attempts within the European Community to begin regulating psychotherapy. It is too early to predict the outcome of either of these initiatives but they seem likely to have some impact on the practice of counselling.

CONCLUSION

The boundaries between counselling skills, counselling and professional roles are no longer matters of abstract interest. For some time, establishing the boundaries between these different roles has been recognized as having important implications for practice. For instance, in health care, there is a need for better ways of classifying the non-medical interventions with patients, especially those designed to offer psychological support. This has become all the more important because of evidence that a good mental attitude accelerates physical recovery. It is appropriate to expect the occupational therapist, nurse, doctor and other health workers to receive training in counselling skills to enhance the quality of their communications with patients. These skills are very useful when listening to a patient's worries or helping a patient decide between treatments. Similarly, all teachers would benefit from a training in counselling skills to help them work with students individually and in seminars and group discussions.

The same observation could be made about so many of the caring professions, from the housing officer dealing with a recently bereaved tenant, the personnel manager working with someone being redeployed, to the social worker with someone reporting suspected sexual abuse, and many other situations. A sound training in counselling skills helps the caring professional to work sensitively with someone's concerns and maintain a sense of whose agenda is being addressed: that of the worker or that of the service user.

However, it is unrealistic to expect all members of the caring professions to train or work as counsellors. The training would be too time-consuming and expensive for all workers in the caring professions. Also, it would be inappropriate for some workers to combine their primary role with that of being a counsellor as this could compromise their professional role, particularly if that requires taking responsibility for someone or having authority over them. Taking on the role of counsellor requires the opportunity to respect the client's capacity for self-determination, even if this is within limits agreed between the counsellor and client. Maintaining this distinction between the 'use of counselling skills' and 'counselling' has helped to clarify the resource implications of each role and created clearer thinking by managers, workers and clients where this distinction is maintained.

The concept of counselling as a contracted role with specific clients rather than an all-embracing title for everything done by someone with the occupational title of counsellor has opened up the possibility of someone taking on several roles so long as they are able to communicate clearly what these roles are and clarify the expectations of service users about the role being undertaken by the helper.

The overall effect of these distinctions between roles is liberating and clarifying for the caring professions. Some fear that instead of freeing up the provision of counselling, the clarification of roles will lead to the increasing regulation of counselling. Certainly this is a possible outcome. The challenge will be to cope with the inevitable increasing regulation of counselling and other caring roles without destroying their responsiveness to potential users of their services. It will be particularly important with counselling to avoid claiming so much professional mystique that counselling no longer rests on foundations of respect for the client's values, personal resources and capacity for self-determination.

REFERENCES

Argyle, M. (ed.) (1981) *Social Skills and Health*, Methuen, London.

Bond, T. (1989) Towards defining the role of counselling skills, *Counselling, the Journal of the British Association for Counselling*, **69**, 3–9.

Bond, T. (1991) *HIV Counselling. Report on National Survey and Consultation*, British Association for Counselling, Rugby.

Breakwell, G.M. (1987) A survey of student counselling in higher and further education in the United Kingdom, *British Journal of Guidance and Counselling*, **15**, no. 3, 285–96.

British Association for Counselling (1985) *Counselling:Definition of terms in use with expansion and rationale*, BAC, Rugby.

British Association for Counselling (1989) *Code of Ethics and Practice for Counselling Skills*, BAC, Rugby.

British Association for Counselling (1990) *Code of Ethics and Practice for Counsellors*, BAC, Rugby.

Gustad, J.W. (1953) The definition of counselling, In R.F. Berdie (ed.) *Roles and Relationships in Counselling*, University of Minnesota Press, Minneapolis.

Ivey, A. and Simek-Downing, L. (1980) *Counselling and Psychotherapy: Skills, theories and practice*, Prentice Hall, New Jersey.

Pashley, B.W. (1976) The life (and death?) of a student counselling service, *British Journal of Guidance and Counselling*, **4**, no. 1, 49–58.

Pratt, J. (1990) The meaning of counselling skills, *Counselling, the Journal of the British Association for Counselling*, **1**, no. 1, 21–2.

Roberts, R. and Fallowfield, L. (1990) The goals of cancer counsellors, *Counselling, the Journal of the British Association for Counselling*, **1**, no. 3, 88–91.

Sykes J.S. (1982) *The Concise Oxford Dictionary*, Oxford University Press, Oxford.

2

Supervision

Ian Horton

By its very nature, helping people cope with psychological problems makes considerable emotional demands upon health professionals. Supervision is intended to help overcome some of these difficulties and provide the opportunity for practitioners to monitor and develop their effectiveness.

Supervision is now widely acknowledged as a basic component of counsellor education and training (Dryden and Thorne, 1991; BAC, 1990a). Indeed, any practitioner who uses some form of counselling as a way of responding to the needs of their patients or clients should continue in supervision (BAC, 1990b). One of the arguments for ongoing supervision is that the practitioner is not always aware of what is going on in their relationship with the client. There may be some part of the practitioner's experience and feelings that remains hidden below the surface or on the edge of awareness (Gendlin, 1984). While what might be called 'unconscious experience' is the central focus in some theories of counselling (e.g. psychodynamic), even within the person-centred tradition it is believed that hidden feelings may influence our behaviour and be completely independent of our conscious awareness (Greenberg and Safran, 1987, p. 47). Only through working with someone else, as in supervision, can a practitioner become aware of these feelings or sensations and the way in which they may affect the relationship and the counselling process. Perhaps Ekstein and Wallerstein (1972) get at the nub of supervision when they say it is about becoming aware of our dumb spots – things we don't know or can't do; our blind spots – our own covert fears, prejudices and pre-occupations; and our deaf spots – things we have repressed or do not want to hear about ourselves and our work. If we can be open enough to allow this to happen it can provide one of the most fruitful and productive outcomes of supervision.

However, initial attitudes towards supervision tend to be ambivalent. On the one hand, supervisees are pleased or even relieved to know that they will receive support and guidance on what concerns them most about their work with clients. It can be a really good feeling to know that you are not working alone and that you can readily seek advice and talk to your supervisor about what has been going on and discuss what to do next. On the other hand, they tend to feel apprehensive or threatened by what they see as exposing their professional competence to the scrutiny and possible criticism of others.

Perhaps the word 'supervision' is unhelpful in this context. It can imply subordination, control, direction and authority to inspect: if a person needs supervision then they cannot be sufficiently competent to work on their own. However, a more positive and self-empowering view is to approach supervision as a way of achieving SUPER-vision for yourself (Houston, 1990). So, rather than seeing the supervisor as a purveyor of superior vision and supervision as something which is done to you, it is possible to see it as something *you* do, an opportunity and resource to develop your own thinking, way of working, and effectiveness.

The practitioner is a participant, not a recipient. It is important for the practitioner to avoid a pupil-teacher role relationship and not simply sit back and wait for the supervisor to make it happen. Hawkins and Shohet (1989, p. 28) warn that 'it is all too easy to slide back into dependency and just accept the style and level of supervision offered'.

Proctor (1988) provides a useful list of what she calls the supervisee's responsibilities. The list includes such things as:

- Thinking about the key question(s) and issues you want to present and asking the supervisor for time to deal with them;
- Asking for the type of feedback you want;
- Being aware of your own feelings, and monitoring any tendencies to become defensive and immediately responding to any feedback by justifying and explaining what you

did and why. Perhaps an essential corollary of this is to
adopt one of the principles of receiving feedback and that
is to listen carefully and work to understand any feedback
by paraphrasing to check your perception of what is being
said to you, and to do this before evaluating its usefulness
to you;

- Responding as openly as you can to any requests for further
  information or clarification and becoming increasingly able
  to share your thoughts and feelings;
- Reviewing the feedback you receive as the first step in
  deciding what is useful;
- Using immediacy (Egan, 1986) to confront and initiate discussion with your supervisor of any problematic aspect of
  your relationship or the way you work together. This may
  otherwise block any real opportunity for learning and prevent a relationship from developing in which you feel safe
  enough to talk about difficult aspects of your work.

The rest of this chapter is in three sections: the nature and
purpose of supervision, and preparation for it. An appendix
provides a framework for presenting information during supervision.

NATURE OF SUPERVISION

Supervision is defined here as a formal contractual arrangement
which enables practitioners to discuss their counselling work
with someone who is appropriately experienced in counselling
and supervision. The formality is important. It makes the distinction between supervision which establishes and maintains
ethical boundaries (BAC, 1990b) and what may otherwise happen
in casual conversations with a colleague to let off steam about a
particularly 'difficult client.' Most ethical codes would see this as
inappropriate and a breach of confidentiality. The contractual
arrangement sets up a supervisor–supervisee role relationship
for the duration of the supervision sessions. This helps to separate the activity from other work roles and relationships. The
ideal is to work with a supervisor with whom you have no other
relationship.

The supervisory contract should make explicit such things
as time, place, frequency, length and purpose of supervision
sessions. Supervision needs to be regular and sufficient (BAC,

1990a). What constitutes regular and sufficient will depend on the amount of counselling undertaken and the experience of the practitioner. For example, BAC accredited counsellors are required to undertake a minimum of one and a half hours supervision a month, but beginning practitioners will tend to meet their supervisor much more frequently.

Supervision normally takes place individually or in a small group with one supervisor. The length of sessions is about an hour, with longer for group supervision. Experienced practitioners may at times find peer group or reciprocal peer supervision (Houston, 1990) sufficient to meet their needs. In addition to periodically 'presenting a client' for supervision, beginning practitioners will need to have some form of regular contact with their supervisor every week or fortnight, and during that time to at least have the opportunity to receive brief feedback on any problematic aspect of their work with current clients (BAC, 1990a).

The term 'supervision' is used to describe a heterogeneous set of conditions and activities. These may include such things as: didactic teaching, interpersonal or microskills training, role play, use of audio or video tape recordings of client sessions, discussion of client material and forming hypotheses about core conflicts, mapping out content areas to deal with if change is to take place, together with generating possible alternative strategies and interventions to facilitate change.

Sometimes supervision may blur into personal counselling for the supervisee. Certainly a practitioner's own thoughts and emotions are relevant to supervision in as much as they may be used within the counselling relationship and provide clues to what is going on in the client. Mearns (1988) has written one of the most useful discussions of this kind of phenomenon. His approach is through the person-centred concept of congruence, but he suggests that it might easily translate into the psychoanalytic language of transference and countertransference (Mearns, 1988, p. 95). A practitioner's own life conflicts and issues may be directly restimulated and impinge on the working relationship with a client, and such material may usefully be explored in supervision (Searles, 1955).

It is important, however, that the boundary between personal counselling and supervision should be maintained. Ideally, the practitioner needs to make separate provision for personal counselling or therapeutic support should this become necessary at any stage (BAC, 1984).

The agenda for supervision contains two inter-related dimensions of counselling or interpersonal relationships: content and process. The content is the detail of the client's psychological problem – the client's thoughts, feelings and behaviour. It is concerned with what the client is saying or otherwise communicating, together with theoretical frameworks for assessment and practical interventions for facilitating change. These explanatory frameworks or worldviews help the practitioner make sense of what the client is saying and enable the client to develop new perspectives (Egan, 1986) or more healthy ways of thinking and behaving. Nicolson and Bayne (1990) provide a clear account of an atheoretical process model of counselling derived from Egan and others. It can be used at various levels as a framework to integrate different theoretical models and is therefore applicable to both beginners and experienced practitioners.

The focus on content in supervision is on the topics and issues presented by the client. There are three levels at which the content can be explored. They represent a sequence.

1. *What is the client saying?*
   This is literal description, of what is overt and without explanation or interpretation.
2. *In what way is what the client is saying important to discuss?*
   This is a search for any underlying feelings and the meaning or particular significance for the client of what she or he has said.
3. *What else, not being said by the client, may be important to explore?*
   This develops from level two exploration into facets of the problem the client may have found too painful and at some point chosen to ignore or repress. At this level the practitioner may begin to make connections between topics or incidents and identify patterns of behaviour.

These are fundamental questions about the content of counselling (Gilmore, 1973) and are at the heart of therapeutic listening.

The second dimension is the process of counselling. Again it may be helpful to identify two levels.

1. The first level examines the practitioner's responses, interventions and strategies.

The BAC Code of Ethics and Practice (1990b) states that counsellors need to be able to account for what they do and why they do it. In supervision you may be invited to reflect on what Caskey *et al.* (1984) in their research into the quality and effectiveness of counselling refer to as intention and impact. It is concerned with trying to answer two questions:

(a) What was I trying to accomplish in saying or doing that? (i.e. intention)
(b) What was the effect on the client of that particular intervention? (i.e. impact)

For the more intuitive practitioners it may be especially challenging or even irritating to be asked why, when it just felt right to do or say something, but the argument is that development as a counsellor requires the ability to reflect consciously on why and what you are doing and its effect on the client. Obviously, what you are trying to do as a practitioner will depend on the particular set of basic assumptions and theoretical frameworks on which you base your practice. Working on developing awareness of intention and impact in supervision will help you continually to evaluate and evolve your own style and repertoire of skills and strategies.

2. The second level of the process dimension looks at the developing relationship between the practitioner and client. There are three facets to explore: what is going on within the practitioner; what is going on within the client; and what is going on between them. This level of process involves the predominantly unaware reactions of the client and practitioner, their thoughts and feelings which may be described as at the edge of awareness and brought into sharper focus through reflection in supervision. The aim is to develop insight and understanding of the dynamics of the relationship.

Kagan (1976, p.234) suggests that when two people talk to each other, it is almost inevitable that each has feelings and thoughts, that each perceives the other as having feelings and thoughts, and that each may wish to impress the other in certain

ways. Perhaps it is also inevitable that at some level of awareness as we talk to other people, they may remind us of people
we have known at other times and other places. Kagan further
suggests that there will not be time to say all we want to say;
there will be things we don't want to say; there will be vague
feelings we can't find words for; impressions we have of others
and impressions we think that they have of us. There will be a
continuous flow of thoughts, feelings and physical sensations.

Reflection on this level of the process dimension can help to
retrieve something useful from this wealth of information.
Hawkins and Shohet (1989) have a further mode or level in their
model of supervision. The focus is on what they describe as the
here-and-now process (i.e. supervision) as a mirror or parallel
of the there-and-then process (i.e. counselling). The aim is to
explore the dynamics of the supervisory relationship on the
assumption that it may provide an alternative window onto the
counselling process (Searles, 1955).

PURPOSE OF SUPERVISION

The primary purpose of supervision is to enable practitioners
both to develop and maintain their usefulness to clients. It is a
way of monitoring the quality of their counselling work and
safeguarding the interests of clients.

Most of the literature on supervision identifies various tasks
or supervisory functions (e.g. Kadushin, 1976; Inskipp and
Proctor, 1988; Hawkins and Shohet, 1989). Although they use
slightly different terms, they broadly reflect three core tasks.
These are not separate or distinct ways of working. In practice,
all forms of supervision will need to contain some aspect from
each of the three tasks or functions.

1. *Educational.* Here the main purpose is for practitioners to
   gain a deeper understanding of the content and process and   to
   develop their skills and ability to integrate theory with
   practice. The supervisor functions primarily as a teacher or
   facilitator. In training, supervisors may have a role in
   assessing the level of learning and have some responsibility
   for clients' welfare.
2. *Managerial.* Here the purpose is to organize and evaluate the
   work being done with the client. Supervisees will be

involved in monitoring the effectiveness of their own work. Supervisors, however, will function as administrators and managers and their main responsibility will be for clients' welfare. They will be primarily accountable to their employer or organization. This raises a contentious issue within some organizations where the practitioner's own line manager is also the person who provides supervision. It can create a relationship in which it is very difficult to relax and be open and honest in the role of supervisee. It can set up a pattern of spurious compliance in which practitioners carefully monitor and select what information to present in order to convey a particular impression to their supervisor. This is one of the reasons I previously suggested that your supervisor should be someone outside any existing relationship. Some employers, however, may find it hard to justify the additional resource implications and be concerned about handing over responsibility to, or even threatened by the existence of, an independent supervisor.

3. *Consultative.* Here practitioners use the supervisor as a case consultant. They are largely autonomous and retain responsibility for their work with clients and control of the supervision agenda. Supervisors are primarily accountable to their supervisees. Perhaps the term 'consultant' or 'consulting supervision' may be more accurately descriptive of the task and shift the perceived power base away from the supervisor towards the supervisee.

Educational and managerial functions tend to concentrate power with the supervisor – especially if they include assessment of supervisees' performance. It is this inequality of the perceived 'you are up and I am down' supervisory relationship that can give rise to the fears and anxieties which some people experience when starting supervision (Rioch, 1980, p. 70).

The purpose of supervision, whether it is primarily educational, managerial or consultative, is to provide an appropriate balance of what may be regarded as the universal components of both counselling and all forms of supervisory relationship: support and challenge.

In much the same way as a counsellor needs to be able to contain or hold clients' emotional distress, the supervisor will need to support the practitioner in supervision. Support in supervision involves empathic understanding of the practitioner's own interpersonal struggles, positive feedback for productive interventions, encouragement with the inevitable stress which results from dealing with difficult, suicidal, seductive or manipulative clients, and the restimulation of distressing aspects of the practitioner's own life experience. The essence of support in supervision is in the feeling of being understood by your supervisor and genuinely respected for what you are as a person and what you are trying to do with your clients.

When people start counselling work they often need to feel competent, finding it difficult to tolerate periods of helplessness, not understanding what is going on, not knowing what to say or do and this contributes to their having difficulty in assuming an appropriate professional role identity. They tend to invest heavily in their clients' welfare, in part because doing so gives a sense of importance that their trainee or beginner status may otherwise deny.

Clients are often all too willing to accept advice or even expect someone else to take care of them, while beginning practitioners may try to make up for all the unhappiness their client has experienced. This can easily result in a form of collusion or what Weiner and Kaplan (1980, p. 44) describe as a covert deal between practitioner and client: 'I'll make you feel special and loved, if you get better and make me feel competent and useful'.

Challenge is the other side of supervision. It is the key to learning, to increased self-awareness and to growth as a person and practitioner. In supervision, even the task of having to organize your thoughts and actually present them to someone else can clarify what you really think and what you feel. In an audio-tape on basic counselling skills, Johns (Johns and Inskipp, 1979) reminds us that, 'often you don't know what you think until you hear what you say'. It is in the act of talking about your counselling work, of getting it out of your head and communicating to the supervisor, and by doing so, to yourself, that you begin to challenge your understanding of the client's problem and what you are trying to achieve.

In a book on co-counselling, which is like reciprocal peer supervision in that the counsellor and client exchange roles,

Evison and Horobin (1983, p. 72) use the dimensions of support and challenge to describe the client and counsellor relationship. The four possible types of relationship they describe are directly applicable to the practitioner-supervisor relationship.

1. Low support and low challenge produce boredom and apathy.
2. High support and low challenge may be appropriate on some occasions and, if effective, will almost certainly feel safe, but it can be seductive and there is always the risk of collusion and little motivation to learn.
3. Low support and high challenge may provide a stimulating and productive relationship for some practitioners, especially those confident in themselves and their counselling, but it can be potentially harmful and can push the practitioner into a defensive corner.
4. High support and high challenge provide the necessary ingredients for the most effective supervisory relationship. The practitioner is likely to feel safe and therefore able to accept and respond more openly and fully to challenges.

PREPARATION FOR SUPERVISION

Most practitioners have only one or two hours supervision a month, so it may be helpful to think about how you want to use the time and what you want to get out of the session. This will not only enable you to make full use of the time available but will help you assume a feeling of greater control, of using the supervision to get what you want from it. Identifying a key question or issue you want to work on, for example, helps to determine what material to present and helps the supervisor to know what to listen for and how to respond. It may also avoid time spent on what in retrospect you regard as irrelevant discussion.

It is good practice to make a brief note of any thought or issue as and when it occurs to you. In this way you will have a record of anything you may wish to reflect upon or get some feedback on in supervision. Perhaps include a section labelled 'questions for supervision' in your case notes.

Some practitioners tend to feel more confident if they use some form of aide-memoire in supervision. This may take the form of your usual case notes or notes written specially for supervision. Audio-tape recordings of your counselling provide a lot of potentially valuable material for micro-analysis and a powerful stimulus for reflection. It is less likely to be so readily filtered by your own perceptions and memory of what happened. Recording a session does, of course, raise ethical issues, especially confidentiality, and tends to increase anxieties – not least those of the practitioner. It may feel like having a supervisor sitting there making judgements about your work. Dryden (1983) provides a provocative analysis and some useful advice on how to cope with recording and supervision anxiety.

Achieving for yourself that SUPER-vision of your counselling work does mean being prepared to take risks and talk about aspects of yourself and your work which you may find difficult. It may feel almost like setting yourself up to be judged, or simply risking hearing yourself say what you don't really want to hear. Ekstein and Wallerstein (1972) warn that without taking risks there will be no significant gain. Supervisees pondering on what to present for supervision may well be faced with the dilemma: 'Am I going to look good, or am I going to learn something?' (Rioch *et al.*, 1976, p. 6). The implication is that you are more likely to learn from presenting an aspect of your work about which you feel unsure and which concerns you in some way. Occasionally, though, we all need to present work which we feel is going well and reflects our level of competence.

What and how you present will depend on what you want to achieve. If your main concern is feeling stuck with a particular client and wondering how to proceed, it may not be necessary to start by presenting the whole story of your work with the client from the beginning through to the last session. Presenting your work with a client in this way takes time and a lot of the background information will not be relevant. In this instance you might start with the present and work backwards. Together with the supervisor and other group members, build up a picture of the client and what you tried to achieve in the last session. In this way you will not create a situation in which you are tempted to use the 'yes, but I did actually try that and it didn't work' response to any therefore redundant suggestions you receive.

There are several different types of material you might wish to present:

1. *An interpersonal episode.* Such episodes include talking to a patient or patient's family, a difficult exchange with a colleague, speaking up at a staff meeting, and so on.

2. *A particular issue.* Here the focus is not on one particular client but on one specific aspect of your experience working with a number of clients. Some categories and examples:

   (a) Conflict of roles, e.g. as both occupational therapist andcounsellor with the same client.

   (b) Your own expectations or needs – to feel wanted, to be effective, to be kind and understanding (which is ofte nclose to collusion or appeasement), for the client to get better or to do what you know is best.

   (c) Your own fears or experience – dealing with seductive clients, rejection, hostility or disappointment, feeling lost, not knowing what to do, fear of the strength of client feelings getting out of control, self-doubts, help-lessness and incompetence.

   (d) Organizational pressure – for you to get the client to conform, be compliant or behave in a particular way, to prove that counselling is a valid use of resources, to get visible results.

   (e) Client expectations – for you to provide a solution, advice, come up with the right answer and tell them what to do.

   (f) Client behaviour – being silent, reluctant to talk, resis-tant to the whole idea of counselling, crying, non-stop talking, arriving late or too early, telephoning you be-tween sessions, threatening suicide or violence, walk-ing out or not turning up.

   (g) Counselling practice – how to start or finish a session, deciding what to do next, legal or ethical issues, facili-tating referral to another agency or counsellor.

3. *A critical incident analysis.* Here the focus is on a specific episode or problematic incident during a session with one client. The presentation would start with a detailed description of the situation and follow with some analysis of the process dynamics, what was said or not said, what was going on within you, your perception of what might have been going on within the client, and between you and the client. The

description and analysis need to be two separate and distinct steps in reflection.

4. *A particular session.* The focus is more on the interchange of responses and interventions throughout one particular session with a client. It requires, as far as possible, a detailed step-by-step description of who said what and when and how they said it, and would usually need to be based on notes you made soon after the session.

5. *A particular client.* This is the typical training presentation. The focus is on the presentation of your work with one particular client over a series of sessions, and you explore and reflect on the content of client material and the dynamics of the developing relationship.

On some occasions, however, it may be appropriate to arrive for supervision with nothing in your mind, and to use the time to review what has been going on for you. Start by relaxing, concentrate on becoming aware of your breathing and then trust that something will surface when you start talking (Inskipp and Proctor, 1988). Another useful technique is scanning (Ernst and Goodison, 1985). Relax and let your mind drift over your counselling work, think aloud and briefly say whatever comes into your mind, without dwelling on any one client or incident. Do not interpret or analyse – just remember and describe. You may find while scanning that one issue or memory looms larger and stirs up more feelings in you than any other. Contract to work on that.

The appendix on p. 28 provides a framework for presenting a client for supervision. It can be easily adapted for other modes of presentation and some sections (e.g. focus on content, focus on process or critical incident analysis) may be used independently.

It is suggested that generally your first task is to describe the client, how they came to see you, their appearance, etc., and the story of their life as they told it. The aim here is to develop an awareness of what actually took place; to, as Hawkins and Shohet (1989) put it, 'meet the phenomena' and get back to what happened. It is sometimes useful to close your eyes and picture your client sitting in front of you. Describe the person you see, what she or he does and says. It is often difficult to stay with our clients in supervision, difficult to tolerate a period of not knowing what is happening, feeling helpless and incompetent. Our account is often clouded by our own rationale, or filter. It is so easy to miss the obvious in our efforts to search for deep and significant meaning and leap to premature or inappropriate explanations and action in order to feel competent.

The essence of supervision is the development of what Schon (1983) calls the 'reflective practitioner'. It can help develop your own 'internal supervisor' (Casement, 1985) to whom you will then have access while actually working with clients. It can provide a kind of internalized support or selfsupervision which can be practised on your own soon after a counselling session or using an audio-tape to stimulate recall.

APPENDIX

Presenting a client for supervision – some frameworks for supervision and case study.

1. **Identification**
   1.1 A first name only. Gender. Age group/life stage.
   1.2 Your first impressions, physical appearance.

2. **Antecedents**
   2.1 Contact. How the client came to see you, e.g. self-referred.
   2.2 Context/location, e.g. agency, private practice, hospital clinic.
   2.3 Pre-contact information. What you knew about the client before you first met. How you used this information. Any existing relationship or previous contact with the client and possible implications.

3. **Presenting Problem and Contract**
   3.1 Summary of client's presenting problem.
   3.2 Your initial assessment. Duration of problem. Precipitating factors (i.e. why the client came at this point). Current conflicts or issues.
   3.3 Contract. Frequency, length and number of sessions. Initial plan.

4. **Questions for Supervision**
   4.1 Key question(s) or issues you want to discuss in supervision.

5. Focus on Content

5.1 Client's account of problem situation:
  - (a) Work – significant activity, interests. How client spends his/her time and energy.
  - (b) Relationships – significant people, family and friends.
  - (c) Identity – self-concept, feelings and attitudes about self.

  Additional related or explanatory elements might include client's past/early experiences; strengths and resources; beliefs and values; hopes, fears and fantasies. Possible implications of cultural, economic, social, political and other systems.

5.2 Problem definition – (a) Construct a picture of the client's view of the present scenario; (b) What is the client's preferred scenario? What would client like to happen? How would client like things to be? (Egan, 1986).

5.3 Assessment and reformulation – how you account for and explain the presenting problem.
  - (a) Patterns/strands/themes/connections which emerge.
  - (b) In what way are these things important to explore? What theoretical concepts/models or explanatory frameworks for assessment? What hunches, new perspectives?
  - (c) What else, which has not been mentioned, might be important to explore? What silent hypotheses, blind spots? What underlying issues or past problems?

5.4 Counselling plan
  - (a) What direction or focus for future work? What possibilities, agenda?
  - (b) What criteria for change: theoretical frameworks and assumptions?
  - (c) Review and/or formulate plan(s).

6. Focus on Process

6.1 Strategies and interventions
  - (a) What strategies and interventions have you used?
  - (b) What were you trying to achieve?
  - (c) What was the effect on the client?
  - (d) Generate alternative options.

6.2 Relationship
(a) What was happening between you and the client? Describe relationship; reframe relationship; try a metaphor.
(b) What was happening within client (transference)?
(c) What was happening within you (counter-transference)?
(d) What changes within developing relationship over the period being discussed?
(e) Evaluate the 'working alliance'.

6.3 Evaluation
(a) Review process.
(b) Consider alternative tasks, strategies and ways of implementing counselling plan(s).

7. Focus on Parallel Process
7.1 What was happening between you and the supervisor?
7.2 Any parallels. What thoughts, feelings, experiences? Does what was going on in the supervisory relationship tell you anything about what may have been going on between you and the client?

8. Critical Incident Analysis
8.1 Description
(a) What did client say or do at that particular point?
(b) What did you say or do?
(c) How did client respond to your intervention?
(d) What was happening within you?

8.2 Analysis
(a) What was happening within client?
(b) What was going on between you and the client?
(c) Intention and impact of interventions/responses.
(d) What hunches/hypotheses did you/do you have?
(e) Review. Any further/alternative perspectives, strategies and interventions.

9. Listening to Aspects of Covert Communication
9.1 What was happening within you? How well can you listen to your own emotional response to a client? You may be aware of your feelings first and thoughts later. Reflection on your

emotional experience may help you gain information about what part of the client is likely to be in need of change.

A simple way of using yourself as a measuring instrument is to ask:
(a) How does this client make me feel?
(b) What did the client say and do so that I feel the way I do?
(c) What does the client want from me and what sort of feeling is she or he trying to arouse in me to get it?

9.2 What was happening within the client?
Different kinds of listening to pick up on whatever is live and poignant for the client at a particular moment. The emphasis is on aspects of covert experience, rather than explicit content.

You can learn to listen for/observe and reflect back when appropriate:
(a) Changes in voice quality – which might indicate an inner focus on something that is being seen or felt differently.
(b) Highly sensory/idiosyncratic words or phrases.
(c) Aspects of content you don't actually understand – perhaps the client doesn't either.
(d) Encoded statements – about other people or situations which may at some level be about the client with reformulations. For example, client says: 'It upset me to see the little dog was alone'. A reformulation might be: 'Seeing the little dog gave you a sense of desolation and rejection. Something about loneliness worries you' (Rice, 1980, p. 144).

Reformulation to focus on the client can be practised almost as a game in supervision.
(e) Indirect or disguised communication. Anything said about something out there may be about you and /or the counselling relationship. Use immediacy (Egan, 1986).
(f) Non-verbal communication, e.g. silence, gazing into space, posture. Try a hunch about the client's inner experience.

REFERENCES

British Association for Counselling (1984) *Supervision*, Information Sheet 8, BAC, Rugby.

BAC (1990a) *The Recognition of Counsellor Training Courses*, BAC, Rugby.

BAC (1990b) *Code of Ethics and Practice for Counsellors*, BAC, Rugby.

Casement, R. (1985) *On Learning from the Patient*, Tavistock, London.

Caskey, N.H., Barker, C. and Elliott, R. (1984) Dual perspectives; clients' and therapists' perceptions of therapist responses, *British Journal of Clinical Psychology*, **23**, 281–90.

Dryden, W. (1983) Supervision of audio-tapes in counselling: obstacles to trainee learning, *The Counsellor*, **3**, no. 8, 18–25.

Dryden, W. and Thorne, B. (eds.) (1991) *Training and Supervision for Counselling in Action*, Sage, London.

Egan, G. (1986) *The Skilled Helper*, 3rd edn, Brooks-Cole, California.

Ekstein, R. and Wallerstein, R.W. (1972) *The Teaching and Learning of Psychotherapy*, International Universities Press, New York.

Ernst, S. and Goodison, L. (1985) *In Our Own Hands*, Women's Press, London.

Evison, R. and Horobin, R. (1983) *How to Change Yourself and Your World*, Co-Counselling Phoenix, Sheffield.

Gendlin, E.T. (1984) The client's client; the edge of awareness, in R.F. Levant and J.M. Shlien (eds.) *Client Centred Therapy and the Person-Centred Approach*, Praeger, New York.

Gilmore, S.K. (1973) *The Counsellor-in-training*, Prentice Hall, London.

Greenberg, L.S. and Safran, J.D. (1987) *Emotion in Psychotherapy*, Guildford, London.

Hawkins, P. and Shohet, R. (1989) *Supervision in the Helping Professions*, Open University Press, Milton Keynes.

Houston, G. (1990) *Supervision and Counselling*, Rochester Foundation, London.

Inskipp, F. and Proctor, B. (1988) *Skills for Supervision and Being Supervised; Audio Tape 1 Booklet: Being Supervised*, Alexia Publications, St Leonards on Sea.

Johns, H. and Inskipp, F. (1979) *Principles of Counselling: Series 1 Audio Tapes Unit 1*, Alexia Publications, St Leonards on Sea.

Kadushin, A. (1976) *Supervision in Social Work*, Columbia University Press, New York.

Kagan, N. (1976) *Interpersonal Process Recall: A method of influencing human interaction*, Office of Medical Education, Research and Development, Michigan State University.

Mearns, D. (1988) *Person Centred Counselling in Action*, Sage, London.

Nicolson P. and Bayne, R. (1990) *Applied Psychology for Social Workers*, 2nd edn, Macmillan, London.

Proctor, B. (1988) *Supervision on the Working Alliance* (Video Tape Training Manual), Alexia Publications, St Leonards on Sea.

Rice, L.N. (1980) A client centred approach to supervision, in A.K. Hess (ed.) *Psychotherapy Supervision: Theory, research and practice*, Wiley, New York.

Rioch, M.J. (1980) The dilemmas of supervision in dynamic psychotherapy, in A.K. Hess (ed.) *Psychotherapy Supervision: Theory, research and practice*, Wiley, New York.

Rioch, M.J., Coulter, W.R. and Weinberger, D.M. (1976) *Dialogues for Therapists*, Jossey Bass, San Francisco.

Schon, D.A. (1983) *The Reflective Practitioner: How professionals think in action*, Temple Smith, London.

Searles, H.F. (1955) The information value of the supervisor's emotional experience, in H.F. Searles (ed.) *Collected Papers on Schizophrenia and Related Subjects*, Hogarth, London.

Weiner, I.B. and Kaplan, R.G. (1980) From classroom to clinic, in A.K. Hess (ed.) *Psychotherapy Supervision: Theory, research and practice*, Wiley, New York.

3

Psychological type, conversations and counselling

Rowan Bayne

This chapter is an introduction to Myers' psychological type theory, in particular its applications to conversations of all kinds, from informal chats to counselling. I discuss:

1. the role of self-awareness in improving conversations;
2. psychological type as an approach to self-awareness and to understanding others, touching on the main concepts and on evidence for their validity; and
3. some applications of type to conversations, counselling and counsellor training.

Finally, there is a brief section on strategies for observing psychological type accurately, and an appendix of guidelines for checking such observations.

CONVERSATIONS AND SELF-AWARENESS

Ideally, the numerous conversations which all health professionals have with clients and colleagues would end with each person feeling listened to and understood. There would be a 'meeting of minds', good communication, true contact. Of course, in practice this happens sometimes and to varying extents – you may like to think for a moment of a conversation that went well, and one that was frustrating, and consider the effects of each conversation on you, on the other people and, if appropriate, on your organization.

Three senses of the term 'self-awareness' are relevant to improving conversations. I have called them inner self-awareness, self-knowledge, and outer self-awareness.

Inner self-awareness refers to thoughts, feelings, etc. A model is outlined in Table 3.1, together with its implications for communicating more fully. You might like to use Table 3.1 to analyse a particular conversation. How many of the elements were spoken, and how precisely and fully? Would any of the unexpressed elements have been relevant and helpful, or not?

I am not suggesting total honesty or unflinching bluntness but fuller expression with some people in some conversations, and a balance of appropriate disclosure and listening. A parallel is with the idea (and fact) that no-one is assertive all the time. Greater self-awareness in the inner, process sense also means a correspondingly greater ability to separate yourself from the other person's views, problems, emotions, etc. and therefore to reduce your chances of misunderstanding them (and they, you). Other possible benefits include noticing signs of stress early and thus having the option of doing something about them early too, and making better decisions.

Self-knowledge – the second sense of self-awareness – refers to relatively stable aspects of inner self-awareness. Thus, if you tend to feel sympathetic more often than antagonistic you might be described as a gentle or caring 'kind of person'. When we ask 'What is she really like?' or 'What sort of person is he?' we are asking about this aspect of self. It too can be included to good effect in some conversations. For example, in discussing a decision with someone, you might say something about your values, interests or personality.

Table 3.1 *Relationships between elements of inner self-awareness and conversation (adapted from Miller et al., 1975. See also Burnard, 1991)*

Awareness of:	Can be disclosed as:
Intentions	I plan to ... I want to ... I'd like to ... etc.
Thoughts	I think ... I wonder ... etc.
Feelings*	I feel ... I am ... etc.
Sensings	I see ... I hear ... etc.

*In this model, the term 'feelings' refers to emotions. In psychological type theory, it has a related but different meaning.

The third sense is outer self-awareness: awareness of how you behave, and of how you appear to other people. It is an obvious part of reflecting on oneself and developing as a practitioner and person, and is the *main* focus (wrongly, in my view) of some courses on self-awareness. However, it too can improve communication, for example by noticing that you are smiling inappropriately or fidgeting, and saying so or stopping or both.

Counsellor training usually assumes that effective counsellors need adequate self-awareness in all three senses, and that this is a life-long process – partly because of its great difficulty and partly because we change. Consider, for example, your current feelings, values and thoughts about death, sex, love, illness, race, ageing – examining them, working through them, coming to terms with them, and how much they have changed in your life so far.

PSYCHOLOGICAL TYPE

Miller *et al.* (1975) suggest that most people have a favourite aspect of inner self-awareness (of those in Table 3.1), one that we are particularly aware of and most able to express well in conversations. Psychological type (Myers, 1980) embodies a similar idea, which overlaps to some extent with their model. The rest of this chapter discusses psychological type and suggests applications to improving and understanding conversations, and particularly to counselling and counsellor training.

Psychological type is Myers' (1980) clarification and development of parts of Jung's theory of personality. She suggested 16 'kinds of people', describing all 16 primarily in terms of strengths and potential strengths. This positive bias is intended to focus and confirm – sometimes to reframe – a person's concept of herself or himself. It is also intended to improve communication and understanding between the types, the general notion here being that if we think about someone who is very different from us in terms of their psychological type, we will be more likely to judge them as different rather than as, say, weird or incompetent.

The central concept is preference, which means 'feeling most comfortable and natural with'. An exercise provides a useful analogy. Please sign your name, first as you usually do and then with your other hand. What is the difference? Generally, your usual hand feels more comfortable, easy and 'natural' while the other takes more effort and feels relatively clumsy and sometimes, as one person put it, 'wobbly'.

Type theory suggests that the four most general ways in which people differ in personality are in pairs of opposites – called **preferences** – and that using them is like using your preferred and non-preferred hands. Most people actually use all eight preferences (four pairs) every day, just as we use both hands, but in widely varying amounts and with very different levels of development or skill. Similarly, each person can behave like more than one type of person, though probably not like all 16. However – and this is the key point – we do not do so with equal facility and fulfilment.

There are four pairs of preferences:

Extraversion	(**E**) or Introversion	(**I**)
Sensing	(**S**) or Intuition	(**N**)
Thinking	(**T**) or Feeling	(**F**)
Judging	(**J**) or Perceiving	(**P**)

Table 3.2 gives a general idea of what these terms mean in type theory, and you may like to choose which of each of the pairs of preferences seems to describe you best. The resulting four letters come in 16 possible combinations, e.g. ENFP, ISFJ, and are, provisionally, your psychological type.

When considering each pair of preferences from Table 3.2, please bear in mind the preferred hand/other hand analogy. You may think of yourself (and others may or may not agree) as equally developed in both, but in type theory one of them is

Table 3.2 *Terms which describe in part the four pairs of preferences when they are developed*

E More outgoing and active ..More reflective and reserved	**I**
S More practical and interested in facts and details ...	
More interested in possibilities and an overview	**N**
T More logical and reasoned ...	
More agreeable and appreciative	**F**
J More planning and coming to conclusions ...	
More easy-going and flexible	**P**

more comfortable for you. You may not find choosing between the preferences easy, and even if you do you may be wrong. I thought I was a particular type for over a year, despite a close friend's clear and well-argued disagreement. She was right. For most people the best way of discovering their true type is to complete the questionnaire associated with the theory, the Myers Briggs Type Indicator (MBTI), with careful interpretation of the results (as outlined in the appendix on p. 47). The MBTI is designed to measure preferences, not how developed they are or how skilfully we use them.

Model of development

So far this description of type has been at the level of the four pairs of preferences. However, type theory also contains a model of how personality develops. The term 'developed' in the heading for Table 3.2 means that the preferences are seen as predispositions. In a 'good enough' environment, these are expressed as characteristic experience and behaviour, and because they are expressed more, they develop more fully. Type theory is optimistic in this respect: it assumes that most people's early socialization allows or encourages the development of their true preferences. However, a child who is, say, introverted by predisposition may be brought up to behave extravertedly. When this happens, type theory predicts inner conflict, ranging from 'not feeling right' through anxiety to neurosis.

The term 'developed' also counters the reaction that a four-letter type sounds like a 'box'. Self-definition requires some limits, and those in type suggest certain preferred patterns and recognize some flexibility, e.g. that some developed ISFPs can behave like developed ESFPs, though probably for less time and with more effort.

Type theory has a further layer: the idea that each person has a *dominant* preference and a second or *auxiliary* preference. Thus, good type development means in part being most skilful with one of Sensing, Intuition, Thinking and Feeling – whichever is your true dominant preference – skilful, but a bit less so, with another preference, and adequately skilful with the third and fourth (Myers, 1980; Provost, 1990; Bayne, 1988). Development is seen as taking a long time, with even the most developed person (in this sense) not achieving good type development until middle age.

A useful twist in type theory, which follows from its model of development, is that strengths tend to have corresponding weaknesses and that those weaknesses tend to be the strengths of the *opposite* type. INFPs, for example, tend to be weakest – or least developed – in ESTJ strengths, and vice versa. Hirsh and Kummerow's (1990) descriptions of the 16 types retain the generally positive tone but also include 'potential pitfalls' and 'suggestions for development'. This aspect of type theory is applied later in this chapter, in the section on giving feedback.

Temperament

Although type is quite complicated, one of its strengths is that several simpler levels of description can be useful, the simplest of all being one of the pairs of preferences in isolation. At an intermediate level of complexity, Keirsey and Bates (1973) suggest four 'temperaments', each identified by two preferences. For example, NF includes INFP, INFJ, ENFP and ENFJ. Speculatively, the basic motives listed in Table 3.3 can be suggested (my partial summary and interpretation). Some of these are probably general human characteristics, but *relatively* important for some temperaments, e.g. everyone needs some excitement (SP) and some stability (SJ), but is one of them *more* characteristic of the particular person?

A related table, on temperament and stress, is in Nicolson and Bayne (1990, p. 110).

Evidence

There are four sources of evidence for the validity of the MBTI and therefore type theory. First, there are numerous relation-

Table 3.3 *Temperament and basic motives*

SP Excitement; solving practical problems; freedom (e.g. from planning in detail); fun; variety.
SJ Being responsible and useful; stability; planning in detail.
NT Understanding ideas; developing new methods/theories/models/a grand vision; competence; analysing and criticizing.
NF Self-development; supporting other people; harmony; authenticity.

ships between type, as measured by the MBTI, and choice of occupation. For example, one type is particularly frequent among executives in various countries, another among clergy of various denominations (Myers and McCaulley, 1985). This does not mean that clergy *cannot* behave like executives, or vice versa, but that generally they do not do so as easily or as often.

A problem with the occupations evidence is that it may just describe self-perceptions, or perhaps calculated self-presentations, not personality or behaviour. Of course executives describe themselves as typically logical and decisive! The second kind of evidence counteracts this criticism: observers' ratings of people generally correlate well with the MBTI results of those observed (Myers and McCaulley, 1985).

The third kind of evidence consists of relationships between type or preferences and much more specific behaviour than occupation, e.g. using certain words more frequently, remembering faces better than objects and vice versa, and, more subtly, style of doing something, and motive (rather than doing it or not). More research of this kind will clarify and improve the descriptions of the types, provide useful clues for observing type accurately and refine the theory. For most purposes, it is also the most useful kind of evidence.

The fourth kind of evidence is the strongest so far for the validity of the MBTI. It consists of relationships between the MBTI and other personality measures, and the most thorough and stimulating study was by McCrae and Costa (1989). Their questionnaire, which comes in both a self-report form (like the MBTI) and a ratings by observers form, has been studied much more than the MBTI, and is strongly related both to behaviour and to the MBTI, thereby supporting the MBTI's validity too. Indeed, McCrae and Costa, though generally very critical of type theory and the MBTI, comment that the MBTI descriptions are 'reasonably good' (p. 35).

This convergence is very encouraging for many psychologists interested in personality theory: two questionnaires developed in different traditions and with different methodologies agree closely on four of the five most general ways in which people differ. Where the two approaches differ most is in the tone of the McCrae and Costa descriptions (much less positive than type), use of the term 'type', type theory's greater versatility, and McCrae and Costa's fifth individual difference, which is 'anxiety'. Anxiety is part of type theory (though rather implicit, in keeping with the positive tone) but not of the MBTI or the basic type descriptions.

TYPE AND COUNSELLING

Type theory and the MBTI are relevant to counselling and counsellor training in four main ways:

- By making concepts like empathy more tangible;
- To analyse and develop counselling skills;
- As a counselling technique;
- As a perspective on counselling practice and on other counselling theories.

Empathy

Type and temperament theory illustrate in a concrete way how difficult it is to be empathic. An ISFP counsellor, for example, is asked to understand (empathize with) an ENFP who she finds rather vague and general, or an INTJ who is most interested in reasons. Psychological contact is easier if she knows that ENFPs and INTJs are on the whole not interested in the same things as she is, and that these are normal and (for them) particularly fulfilling ways to be most of the time.

Type and temperament theory can be used to speed up and deepen empathy. For example, listening to an SJ client talk about pressure of work, I knew from temperament theory that responsibility and conscientiousness were likely to be very prominent in her life and I tried those words with her. If I had not known (or guessed) that she was a developed SJ, or if I had not known that some people are SJs and that I am not, then I would probably have taken longer to understand this quality in the client, or failed to appreciate it at all, or even have challenged it as an *intrinsically* unfulfilling way to be. Some SJs are too conscientious for their own health and effectiveness and could usefully consider developing their P qualities but – according to temperament and type theory – they will always be basically conscientious. If so, then challenging the quality itself – rather than the overuse of it – is futile at best.

Analysing and developing counselling skills

Type provides a language for giving and receiving feedback in a less threatening, more constructive way. It counteracts the tendency of counsellors (and others) to be too hard on themselves, and encourages them to discuss their strengths as well as aspects of their counselling that they need to work on. Perhaps most important, it is a useful counter to myths about 'the good counsellor' or 'the best way to counsel'.

Table 3.4 illustrates these aspects of type and counselling. It also applies the twist described earlier. It lists each preference with (if sufficiently developed) the associated strengths, and (if the opposed preference is not sufficiently developed) aspects to work on. Table 3.4 is experimental but the rationale is clear and a more complicated version has been used successfully in the USA with nursing and medical students (Heinrich and Pfeiffer, 1989).

The main general principle is to build on strengths: in other words, to develop and confirm your type's strengths first and most, and then to *add* to a lesser extent the strengths of the other preferences. For example, counsellors with a preference for, and good development of, S will (a) tend to observe non-verbal communication particularly well but (b) tend to overlook or forget themes or the 'general picture'. According to type theory, they should continue to do (a) well and occasionally remind themselves to check (b).

The counselling terms used in Table 3.4, e.g. paraphrasing and challenging, are in quite general use (though with some variations of meaning); see for example, Nicolson and Bayne (1990, Chapter 3); Egan (1975/1990).

Type as a counselling technique

Type is used in a variety of forms of counselling, e.g. careers, relationship, and various approaches or schools. Type itself includes both a more psychodynamic school (e.g. Quenk and Quenk, 1984) and a more humanistic one (e.g. Provost, 1984). In both schools, the general strategy is to start by helping the client decide on her or his true type, usually by using MBTI results as a starting point. This can be very confirming and hopeful, with problems being 'reframed' as less preferred as-

Table 3.4 *The preferences and aspects of counselling (from Bayne, 1992)*

Likely strengths	Likely aspects to work on
E Helping the client explore a wide range of issues Easy initial contact Thinking 'on feet'	Paraphrasing more Using silence Helping client explore issues in sufficient depth Reaching the action stage too early
I Helping the client explore a few issues in depth Reflecting on strategies, etc. Using silence	Paraphrasing more Helping the client move to action Helping client explore all relevant issues Ease of initial contact
S Observing details Being realistic Helping client decide on practical action plans	Taking the overall picture into account Brainstorming (strategies, challenges and actions) Using hunches
N Seeing the overall picture Brainstorming Using hunches	Being specific Testing hunches Helping client decide on practical action plans
T Being objective Challenging (i.e. from counsellor's frame of reference)	'Picking up' feelings Being empathic (i.e. from client's frame of reference) Being warmer Challenging too early
F Being warm Being empathic	Taking thoughts into account as well as feelings Coping with conflict and 'negative' feelings Being more objective Challenging
J Being organized Being decisive	Helping client to make decisions (i.e. not prematurely) Being flexible
P Being spontaneous Being flexible	Being organized, e.g. keeping to time, structure of session Helping client to make decisions

pects of a person, or as conflicts between preferences, or as qualities to develop.

It is usually most appropriate to use the MBTI (or parts of the theory) as a new perspective, i.e. after the client has explored one or more problems sufficiently and feels understood. If the MBTI itself is used, then it takes about 30 minutes to complete and score, and at least a further 30 minutes to set the scene for testing and verifying – or not – the results. Specialized brief training is highly desirable (addresses at end of chapter).

Perspectives on counselling

Type has implications for counselling itself and for counsellor training. For example, the theory suggests that Thinking types may not be being defensive or intellectualizing when they avoid feelings and emphasize thoughts and reasons. Rather, they may be behaving like developed Thinking types. At some point it may well be helpful for them to clarify their values and feelings but not necessarily from the start. Table 3.5 suggests problems and strategies of communication between each of the pairs of preferences. The table needs qualifying: (1) Conflicts do sometimes occur between people with the same preferences; (2) Some conflicts are nothing to do with type; (3) Opposites are sometimes a powerful attraction – the other person is developed where we would like to be – and sometimes a frustration – the other person is developed in a way we find difficult or worse.

Finally, there is the issue of matching counsellors and orientation, and counsellors and clients. All the types can be effective counsellors and clients but, according to theory and research findings, each is more likely to be drawn to certain schools and aspects of counselling than others. In addition, there is an overall, quite marked bias among counsellors in general towards Feeling (dealing with people) and Intuition (inferring meanings). Some studies have found that psychoanalytic approaches are more attractive to Judging types, cognitive approaches to Thinking types, and so on (Myers and McCaulley, 1985). This does *not* mean that, for example, Feeling types should avoid training in cognitive counselling; it is more a factor for a counsellor to take into account in choosing her or his specialisms.

Table 3.5 *The preferences, some communication problems and some communication strategies*

1. The most likely problems (according to theory) include:

Between E and I	:	contact *v* time alone
Between S and N	:	details and realism *v* general picture and speculation
Between T and F	:	seen as unsympathetic and critical *v* illogical and too agreeable
Between J and P	:	decisive and planning *v* flexible and changeable

2. Some strategies are:

E →I	Allow time for privacy and to reflect
I →E	Explain need for time, allow for other's need for more interaction
S →N	Overall picture first, with relevant details
N →S	Say a particular idea is half-formed and/or include some detail
T →F	Include effects on people, begin with points of agreement
F →T	Include reasons and consequences, be brief
J →P	Allow for some flexibility in plans, style of working, etc. and the other's need not to be controlled
P →J	Allow for some planning and structure, and for the other's need to control

There are many stimulating ideas on type and counselling waiting to be tested systematically. It seems likely that there are guidelines to be discovered (and perhaps already used implicitly), and that type may be a powerful factor, but quite how powerful remains to be seen. In my view, type's value in increasing the 'core qualities' like empathy is already clear, and its uses in other aspects of counselling are promising.

OBSERVING TYPE ACCURATELY

To apply psychological type well, a person needs to be:

1. aware of their own preferences and the relative development of each;
2. able to observe the preferences accurately;
3. able to adjust their style to the other person's (to some extent).

The first and third aspects were discussed earlier in the chapter. This section focuses on the second aspect: accurate observation. If you know a person well then the indications in Table 3.2 or the Report Form brief descriptions of the 16 types (from CAPT or OPP – addresses at the end of the chapter; in Myers, 1987; appendix in Lawrence, 1982; Provost, 1990, pp.20–21) may be sufficient to judge their type or some of their preferences accurately. If you know two preferences, this leaves only four types to decide between. The rest of this section includes some general suggestions about making accurate judgements of personality, and then some further clues to the preferences.

Behaviour is often ambiguous. What we see are clues and evidence, not type or preferences. Accurate judgements of them are made more likely by accepting this intellectually and emotionally, and trying therefore to gather sufficient good evidence for a judgement (Nicolson and Bayne, 1990, Chapter 5). A further precaution is to try to take account of situational pressures including roles and the effects of yourself as the observer. The ideal evidence would be a broad, representative sample of behaviour gathered by skilful observers over a long period and in a variety of situations. In practice, accurate judgements can be made without the ideal conditions because most people behave most of the time like their own type. They also find it more tiring to behave in other ways, and especially to sustain them – a key point of the theory. Given this general starting position, accurate observation of type is possible (cf, McCrae and Costa, 1989) and sometimes more practical than asking people to complete the MBTI.

The EI preference is indicated by where the person's interest 'goes' most easily – outwards or inwards, in action or reflection? There are some simple but not magical tests; for instance, ask an unexpected and novel question, i.e.novel to the person being asked. In theory, Es will tend to answer at once, Is to pause and reflect. Another strategy is to ask yourself, 'How well do I know this person'?, allowing for time spent with them. Es may be easier to get to know than Is.

The JP preference should be relatively visible because it influences how we deal with the 'outside world'. Does the person organize easily, like to get on with things and get them done (J)? Like to keep gathering information (P)? Become quickly bored with routine (P)? Behave in an easygoing way (most of the time) (P)?

Choice of films and books (and style of and motives for reading) can be useful clues to SN; Ss tend to prefer more realistic books and to remember plots and details. For TF, the most obvious strategy is to ask the person to give their reasons for a decision, or to analyse a problem. Ts tend to present more reasons (which may include feelings) and answer in a logical and precise way, Fs to say it felt right and to take more account of effects on other people.

The checklist in Lawrence (1982, pp.69-77, simplified in Bayne, 1988, Figure 1) has been used – apparently with success – in training sales people who are in long term relationships with their prospective buyers to observe their type. Temperament – SP, SJ, NT or NF – should be more observable (it is a theory of behaviour not preference) and useful as a check on judgements of some of the preferences as well as in its own right.

APPENDIX: SOME GUIDELINES FOR INTERPRETING MBTI RESULTS AND OBSERVATIONS OF BEHAVIOUR

Psychological type theory is mainly used to encourage (a) realistic and positive self-awareness and (b) greater understanding of people who are very different 'types'.

Accurate observations and/or skilful interpretation of MBTI results makes achieving these aims more likely. Some guidelines:

1. If the MBTI was completed, it can be helpful to discuss what it was like to do this and, if appropriate, factors such as:
    *   the intrinsic crudeness of personality questionnaires (people interpret questions differently, various biases operate, etc.);
    *   people differ in other important respects (academic ability, anxiety, etc.) but the MBTI does not measure these;
    *   people's *behaviour* is affected by moods, roles, situations, other personality characteristics, how developed each preference is, etc. as well as by their psychological type;
    *   type theory is a theory of personality development, but the MBTI does not measure development or maturity at all;

- all types are valuable. There are no good or bad, sick or well, types/MBTI results.

2. The handedness exercise – writing your signature with your non-preferred hand and then your preferred one, and comparing how the two felt – is a useful analogy with preference and   type.
3. It is important to 'set the scene' for someone to decide (if they want to) what their own type is, in their own time. Observations and MBTI results are a starting point. Other strategies include:

   - asking close friends and relatives about aspects of your-self. The observation checklist in Lawrence (1982, pages 69–77) is a way of doing this;
   - observing your own experience and behaviour closely and systematically, including comparing yourself with others who are clear about *their* own type;
   - carrying out a biographical review or interview, e.g. exploring environmental/social pressures and their possible effects on reported type, and looking for direct early indications of true preference, e.g. an interest (and the way it is spoken about now). Look, too, for a sense of what feels natural and what has been learned with more difficulty (and even as a painful necessity).

   One or more of these strategies can be part of any interpre-tation.

4. The standard framework for an interpretation is to use the 16 sketches on the Report Form (available from CAPT   (USA) and OPP (UK)) before longer descriptions. The person looks for the best fit of the sketches, rather than a perfect fit. The *worst* fit can also be a useful indication. Two qualifications:
   a) The descriptions apply best to people who have devel-oped their dominant function most and their auxiliary function second most, both to a 'reasonable degree'.
   b) The descriptions suggest *likely* behaviour (for the rea-sons noted in point a) and behaviour which tends to be most natural, fulfilling and skilful.

Finally, longer descriptions can be used and discussed, again looking for the best fit, e.g. Myers (1987) and Hirsh and Kummerow (1990).

REFERENCES

Bayne, R. (1988) Psychological type as a model of personality development, *British Journal of Guidance and Counselling*, **16**, no. 2, 167–75.

Bayne, R. (1992) The preferences and aspects of counselling, *Bulletin of Psychological Type*, **15**, no. 1, 14–15.

Burnard, P. (1991) *Coping with Stress in the Health Professions: A practical guide*, Chapman and Hall, London.

Egan, G. (1975/1990) *The Skilled Helper*, 1st and 4th edns, Brooks/Cole, California.

Heinrich, K.T. and Pfeiffer, C.A. (1989) *Using the MBTI to personalise the teaching of interviewing skills*. Paper presented at the biennial international conference of the Association for Psychological Type, University of Colorado, Boulder.

Hirsh, S.K. and Kummerow, J. (1990) *Introduction to Type in Organizations*, 2nd edn, Consulting Psychologists Press, California.

Keirsey, D. and Bates, M. (1978) *Please Understand Me*, 3rd edn, Prometheus Nemesis, California.

Lawrence, G. (1982) *People Types and Tiger Stripes: A practical guide to learning styles*, 2nd edn, Center for Applications of Psychological Type, Gainesville.

McCrae, R.R. and Costa, P.T. (1989) Reinterpreting the Myers-Briggs Type Indicator from the perspective of the five factor model of personality, *Journal of Personality*. **57**, 17–40.

Miller, S., Nunnally, E.W. and Wackman, D.E. (1975) *Alive and Aware: How to improve your relationships through better communication*, Interpersonal Communication Programs Inc., Minneapolis.

Myers, I.B. (1980) *Gifts Differing*, Consulting Psychologists Press, California.

Myers, I.B. (1987) *Introduction to Type*, Consulting Psychologists Press, California.

Myers, I.B. and McCaulley, M. (1985) *Manual: A guide to the development and use of the Myers-Briggs Type Indicator*, Consulting Psychologists Press, California.

Nicolson, P. and Bayne, R. (1990) *Applied Psychology for Social Workers*, 2nd edn, Macmillan, London.

Provost, J.A. (1984) *A Casebook: Applications of the Myers-Briggs Type Indicator in counselling*, Center for Applications of Psychological Type, Gainesville.

Provost, J.A. (1990) *Work, Play and Type*, Consulting Psychologists Press, California.

Quenk, A.T. and Quenk, N.L. (1984) The use of psychological typology in analysis, in Stein M. (ed.) *Jungian Analysis*, RKP, London.

ADDRESSES

1. For training and publications in UK:
    Oxford Psychologists Press (OPP)
    Lambourne House
    311–321 Banbury Road
    Oxford 0X2 7JH
    England
    Phone: 0865 510203
    Fax: 0865 310368

2. For training and publications in USA:
    Center for Applications of Psychological Type (CAPT)
    2720 NW 6th Street
    Gainesville
    FL 32609
    USA
    Phone: 800 777–2248

3. Membership organization (UK):
    British Association for Psychological Type (BAPT)
    Emmaus House
    Clifton
    Bristol BS8 4PD
    England
    Phone: 0272 738056

4. Membership organization (USA):
    Association for Psychological Type (APT)
    9140 Ward Parkway
    Kansas City
    MO 64114
    USA
    Phone: 816 444–3500
    Fax: 816 444–0330

4

Working with potential violence

Jan Burns

INTRODUCTION

The incidence of violence and aggression experienced at work by the health professions appears to be on the increase, both in terms of the frequency and the seriousness of the incidents experienced (Owens and Ashcroft, 1985; Breakwell, 1989; Perkins *et al.*, 1991). This may be due to a combination of factors. Certainly, those cases that have hit the media headlines will have raised awareness and helped legitimize the reporting of experiences. Another influence might be a lack of resources, such as specialized, secure accommodation for people who are violently psychiatrically disturbed, or treatment and care being spread over too thin a workforce in terms of numbers, experience and training, so that errors do occur. Perhaps the important point is that it is now being legitimately recognized that the potential for violence and aggression is becoming an everyday hazard for health professionals.

To prevent such incidents occurring in the future it is imperative to analyse past events and implement the lessons learnt. Relevant findings from such research include:

- Inexperienced staff placed in a situation where violence might occur are more likely to be involved in an incident than more experienced members of staff (MacKay, 1987).
- There may be also be a subsample of staff who experience more episodes of violence and aggression than other staff working in the same conditions, with the same training and having had the same years of experience (Rowett, 1986).
- Working in specialties where violence and aggression characterize the client group, e.g. forensic services, does not

always lead to a higher prevalence of incidents. For example, Perkins *et al.*'s study showed that psychologists were more likely to be physically assaulted if they worked in psychiatric rehabilitation, neuropsychiatry and learning disabilities than in the forensic services (Perkins *et al.*, 1991).

THE 'CARING' PROFESSIONS

An issue that is often faced by health professionals is the paradoxical situation of trying to 'care' for somebody who by definition is vulnerable and in need of help, and by so doing placing oneself in a potentially vulnerable position; the client then has a chance to take advantage of the situation and assault the person who 'cares'.

If we construe the carer-client relationship in terms of power, such incidents start to make more sense. The client is usually placed in a position of powerlessness, whilst the professional carer is in a position of power. If for some reason the situation becomes untenable the powerless will take power. Aggression is the most effective way of doing this in this context, and carers are an 'easy', available target. Bound up with caring are allied values such as passivity, trust and respect, all adding to the caring professionals being 'soft' targets for aggression. Thus, the construction of 'being on the same side', held by the carer, might well not be one shared by the client.

For example, in a situation where one might expect great allegiance between the workers and the users of a service, Stout and Thomas (1991), in a study of hostels for battered women, found that at least 20% of the staff working in the hostels surveyed had been physically assaulted whilst on duty. All except one assault had been committed by women or children using the service. Interestingly, it was only the assault committed by the batterer where charges were made.

This chapter aims to illustrate how the application of psychological understanding to behaviour can help to maintain safe standards whilst still facilitating the work of the health professional. The evidence presented above suggests that there are ways of managing the environment and using interpersonal skills to reduce the probability that violence will occur.

DEFINITIONS

Before continuing our discussion of violence in the work place, it is perhaps useful to define exactly what we mean by this term. Violence to staff has been defined in the UK by the Department of Health and Social Security (DHSS) as:

'i. The application of force, severe threat or serious abuse, by members of the public towards people arising out of the course of their work whether or not they are on duty'
and it includes:
'ii. Severe verbal abuse or threat where this is judged likely to turn into actual violence; serious or persistent harassment (including racial or sexual harassment); threat with a weapon; major or minor injury; fatalities.'

(DHSS, 1988)

This is a useful definition for a number of reasons.

1. It covers both actual and *threatened* physical violence. Being placed in a situation of continual fear might well have as many damaging consequences as actually being physically assaulted.
2. It covers both physical and verbal violence.
3. It covers both racial and sexual harassment, which are not commonly acknowledged as violence.
4. It does not just turn attention to violence from the client with whom the worker is involved. It takes the wider brief of 'members of the public'. This is important as we have learnt that it is frequently not the client who may commit the violent act, but their carer, spouse, other relative or child.

Interestingly, this definition does not include violence from other colleagues. Given the evidence from the survey of psychologists (Perkins *et al.*, 1991) and incidents reported in other professions such as the police force and army, this might be an important omission.

To enable a person to take action and avoid a violent incident or indeed deal with the aftermath, there has to be a recognition of what constitutes violence. Definitions such as this help us part of the way. However, at some point human judgement comes into play, and probably the most important phrase in the above definition is '... where this is judged likely to turn into actual violence'.

Each person, in each situation, will have to find a demarcation line where they judge that violence is about to or has just occurred and appropriate action needs to be taken. This judgement will be based upon two things: firstly, the expectations within the job, and secondly, the skills they have to deal with violent situations. Taking the first factor, within any profession there must be an acknowledged level of vocational violence. Thus, within the police force where there is a high level of vocational violence, there is some consensus agreement and training on this issue is commensurate with the number and type of incidents likely to be experienced. In the health professions, it is now becoming recognized and expected that dealing with violence might be part of the job, and training is increasing.

Hence, the rest of this chapter addresses the environmental factors that must be taken into consideration, firstly to prevent an incident occurring, and secondly, to deal with an incident should it occur.

POLICY ON AGGRESSION AND VIOLENCE

Within any working environment it must be a priority to maximize the safety of the workers, and this must be done in the least restrictive way so as to allow them to continue their work as unhindered as possible. To facilitate this and to monitor its effectiveness, it is imperative that these issues are addressed in a policy document written with that service in mind, and made available to all workers. Such a policy legitimizes such issues and allows people to make changes and take precautions within the organizational framework, thus not leaving it up to the individual to run the gauntlet of potential machismo attitudes and complacent routines. Some good examples of policies are contained in the report of the DHSS Advisory Committee on Violence to Staff (MacKay, 1987)

CONSULTING ENVIRONMENT

If clients are to be seen in a consulting room environment there are some simple precautions to abide by:

In the waiting area

Confusion, boredom and anxiety can all lead to outbursts of aggression. Therefore:

1. Ensure that there is somebody to receive the client, tell them where to sit, how long they may have to wait, keep them informed of any changes, etc. This reception area should be easily identifiable and accessible, and specific disabilities should be considered, including physical handicaps and literacy.
2. For many people who may be confused, say through dementia, or who have severe psychiatric problems or learning disabilities, an environment which is busy, noisy, and hectic will induce stress which may lead to a violent outburst. A waiting room that is not a thoroughfare but which can be observed by staff is preferable, with enough informally arranged seats and something to read or look at whilst waiting.
3. Consideration should be given to the mix of clients who will be using the waiting room. It may be useful to have another separate room in which to isolate particularly noisy, behaviourally disturbed clients, or particularly distraught individuals. This might also be an issue when people who are in conflict are being brought together for a meeting, such as estranged couples, foster parents and natural parents.

In the office or consulting room

Most incidents occur when the professional is alone with the client, and the client is known to them. Such circumstances usually occur therefore in consulting situations, e.g. in a clinic or interview room. There are a number of precautions that can very simply reduce risk.

1. Have a developed, detailed and tested strategy to call for assistance or to intervene if concerned on behalf of somebody else. This might involve setting up some sort of alarm system. This could be quite simple, such as a coded message by telephone or might be more technologically

sophisticated such as personal alarms or 'panic' buttons in the offices.

2. Do not see clients on your own out of earshot of assistance, or when you are alone in the building.

3. Make sure all corridors, etc. are well lit. An example from the survey of clinical psychologists illustrates the importance of this:

    'He tried to hug me and I kept my distance with a handshake, but when I opened the door it was to find the corridor in darkness ... Though I told him to stay in the office he followed me along the dark corridor.'

    (Perkins *et al.*, 1991, p. 12)

4. Know who is coming to see you. This may be a difficult issue for some who prefer to see new clients 'cold' and not be influenced by notes. However, general questions could be asked of those who do know the client – 'Do you think it is OK if I see this person on my own?'.

5. Do not leave any potential weapons lying around the office, e.g. letter openers, scissors, needles, etc.

6. Do not have anything displayed with your personal address or telephone number, and consider if you should have your name in the phone book.

7. Arrange the chairs so that both you and your client can get out of the door quickly if needs be. Often people who tend to be violent have a larger area of personal space and find ordinary social distances intrusive and anxiety-provoking (McGurk *et al.*, 1981). So it is as well to be aware of this and provide slightly more space around the individual and arrange the seating to allow for this.

8. Do not have a Yale type lock or a key in the door to your office, as this can easily result in you being locked in and not even being aware of it.

HOME VISITING

The majority of women, and many men, would think twice before knocking on the door of a person whom they might never have met and entering their house, on their own, and then talking about things that the person might find particularly emotive or upsetting. However, health professionals do this every day, behaving as if their professional title throws a cloak of protection around them. Realistically, we know that far from protecting them, their professional title might actually be the cause of an attack (Breakwell, 1989).

Many of the incidents that have been reported have occurred whilst people are out on home visits. It is under these circumstances that the worker is perhaps at their most vulnerable – they might not know the environment they are entering, who will be there, and what will be happening. On home visits control over the environment and circumstances is lost, which leaves the worker exposed. However, there are a number of ways in which the potential for harm can be reduced.

1. Unless you know all the circumstances and feel completely safe, do not go alone; take somebody else with you. In times of stretched resources, this might sound something of an ideal recommendation. However, considered in the context of the loss of resources that might occur through physical injury, burn-out, low morale, and resignation from the profession, to be accompanied can be argued as resources well spent.
2. Find out as much as you can about the circumstances of the visit. This will include the aim of your visit, who else might be there other than the client, the likely reception to your visit, the psychological and/or psychiatric state of the client and those others who might be present, and what has happened on previous similar visits.
3. Make a detailed plan of staff whereabouts and movements, with periodic reporting in to base. This should be backed up with a clear policy about what action should be taken should something unexpected happen.
4. Ensure good communication of information. Files should always be regularly updated thus allowing staff to assess risk on valid and accurate information.

FACING A VIOLENT SITUATION

Prevention is always better than intervention. All the methods described earlier are ways of trying to prevent the staff member from being faced with a violent situation. However, it does sometimes occur that the member of staff finds themselves in a potentially dangerous situation. When this arises two things need to happen.

1. They need to assess accurately the level and type of danger facing them.

This should then affect

2. The intervention decided upon and implemented.

Assessing a violent situation

There are a number of clues called 'setting factors' (Monahan, 1981) which help a person to make an assessment of the risk which they face. Some of these setting factors might be known before entering the situation, others will only be known once in the situation. Such setting factors include:

1. *The history of violence attached to the person.* Those people with a history of violence are more likely to be violent again. Violence is often used as a way of solving a problem or coping in a situation. Those with violent histories have demonstrated that this is a preferred way of dealing with difficult circumstances. Knowing this enables one to predict that under similar circumstances they are more likely to revert to this solution than those individuals with less violent histories.

2. *The influence of alcohol and drugs.* Alcohol and drugs lessen a person's inhibitions; thus they are less likely to be able to sanction and control more primitive impulses, such as aggression. Such influences also affect a person's cognitive ability, making them less amenable to reason.

3. *Interpersonal factors.* In situations where the individual holds a status which has been achieved by dominating others, verbal and physical aggression are common methods used to gain and maintain this status. Thus, the person's identity becomes very closely linked with aggression. Hence, in a situation where the individual's status is under threat, such as a conflict between a dominating husband and a female social worker, he may feel emasculated, i.e. not a real man, if he starts to lose status and so reverts to aggression as a way of re-asserting his dominant status, regardless of the content of the conflict.

These dynamics have even more power over people's behaviour when they occur in front of other people. In the above example, if the conflict with the social worker occurred in front of the wife, the husband may feel that his position is even more compromised and react even more quickly to prevent 'losing face'. Peer and social approval are also strong forces that have led many people to do things that ordinarily they may never have done on their own.

4. *Options available.* There is a variety of theories about aggression but an element that is common to many such theories is that it is a response that allows escape from an unpleasant situation (Bandura, 1973). Such unpleasantness may be physical or psychological. Emotions that have for many years been tied closely to aggression are frustration and fear (Dollard *et al.*, 1939). These are in themselves unpleasant feelings, and violence is one way of reducing such feelings. If a person has learnt or knows no other ways of lessening the unpleasantness of a situation then they may feel they have no option but to use violence as a quick, and often efficient, way of escaping.

Hence, it becomes easier to predict that if certain emotions are present such as frustration or fear, combined with a lack of social skills to alleviate such unpleasant feelings, a person is likely to feel that they have no other option open to them but to be violent. If the person experiences positive outcomes to being violent then this action becomes reinforced and more generally used.

5. *Physiological factors.* Violence occurs when a person is physiologically aroused; however, the change from a state of relaxation and passivity to arousal might be very rapid and the observable components of arousal are not always easily detectable and may differ from one individual to the next. Hence, how the person looks is not always an easy predictor of violence. Some people may become very red in the face and tremble, whilst others may turn white and be very still. The important thing to notice is *the change in appearance* as this will indicate some change in physiological arousal. Placing this in the context of what has just occurred or been said will help to predict the build-up towards violence.

6. *Behavioural factors.* Shouting, being aggressive to objects, tense, unpredictable movements, facial expression, staring, clenching of fists, etc. are all clear indicators that the individual is moving towards a state where they might become violent. Again, all these factors are dependent upon what is normal behaviour for that person, and the really

important feature to watch out for is a change in their
normal behaviour.

7. *Cognitive factors*. One of the clearest predictors of violence is
if a person says they are going to be violent. The voicing of
intent may be seen as a threat with the intention to control
or manipulate the situation, but it may also be seen as a
warning, i.e. that the situation is becoming so unbearable
that the person is about to take swift and violent aversive
action unless something changes. Many assaults are not
preplanned, premeditated events, but instances where
control is lost and impulses are acted upon. Intent to harm
may be verbalized in both cases, but in the latter the
motivation for this might be more to warn the potential
victim and so provoke some sort of intervention to avoid
violence. Therefore, it is important to listen to the client and
take such threats seriously.

There is no clear formula by which to predict the risk of
violence occurring. Every situation has to be judged individually, but the setting factors described above should give some
guidance on how such an assessment can be made.

Intervention

Once the situation has been assessed as one of potential violence, a plan of intervention can be decided upon.

1. *Escape*. The first option must always be avoidance. If you can
physically remove yourself and whoever else is at risk, then
do so.

2. *Assuming control and providing other options*. Prior to the
situation erupting there may still be a chance for the
worker to take responsibility and defuse the situation.
Going back to the theory that much violence results
from a desire to curtail unpleasant feelings, and violence
is seen as the only way of doing that, other options might
be offered to reduce this unpleasantness. For example,
one might acknowledge the rising emotions and provide
a safe way to escape from these emotions by perhaps
ending the interview or visit. This must be done without
appearing dismissive or clearly frightened, but in a calm
and confident manner.

3. *Distraction.* This is any method by which the perpetrator is temporarily distracted from carrying out harmful intentions. This might include behavioural distractions such as saying you need to go to the toilet, need to check a door, offer to make a drink, etc. Or they might include more psychological methods such as encouraging the person to talk. This might be about something other than the topic which has aroused them, but in which they have a clear interest.

4. *Mood matching.* This is a controversial technique that is sometimes useful and at other times definitely not useful. The technique suggests that the potential victim matches the mood of the potential assailant, so if they are angry and shouting the victim is angry and shouts; likewise, if they are calm and purposeful the victim is also calm and purposeful. It is easy to understand, even in our own domestic circumstances, that if a person directs anger at another and that other continues to remain very calm, the person feeling angry will become increasingly frustrated and anger will heighten. However, an emotional or aggressive response might also reinforce the assailant's behaviour, increase the demand for them to dominate and be in control, and so increase the likelihood of violence (Forgas, 1985).

5. *Personalization.* This is the technique of building up a personal identity with the aggressor. The theory is that somebody is less likely to commit violence to a person who they see as an individual. However, there may be instances where 'depersonalization' is more useful. For example, in a situation where your assailant wants you to take some action, such as hand over money, information, etc., it may be better to place the responsibility and power on the organization, emphasizing your powerlessness to provide what the attacker wants.

However, under different circumstances, where perhaps you have been chosen not because of who you are but because you symbolize something, e.g. a social worker, it might be better to personalize yourself. This can be done by giving personal information about yourself, e.g. your name, family details, etc., emphasizing your personal and not your professional identity.

Empathizing with the problems of the assailant is a useful technique as it reduces the distance between you and him or her; however, it should be used sensitively as each person feels in some way that their problems are unique to themselves and to say something like 'I know just how you feel' is only likely to inflame the situation.

6. *Non-verbal behaviour.* Again, this is important in aggressive situations. As mentioned earlier the aggressive person is likely to have a larger body space around them than the average person (McGurk *et al.*, 1981) so you need to keep physically further away. Stand or sit in a posture that is non-confrontational, e.g. at 45 degrees rather than head-on, and avoid prolonged eye contact as this might increase the aggression (Argyle, 1984). Do not turn your back, and do not draw your assailant's attention to possible weapons by trying to remove them in their sight.

7. *Bystander intervention.* The apathy of bystanders about intervening in violent situations is now a well-known social psychological phenomenon. If you are in a situation where bystanders are looking on, Breakwell (1989) suggests that there are two things to do to break this apathy:

   (a) Identify one person to direct your attention to;
   (b) Make a clear and specific request for help to that person, e.g. 'Go and ring the police from that shop over there', not just 'Go and get help'.

Whatever the setting factors, each situation has to be judged on its own merits, but there are two factors which may assist in making the right decisions:

1. Clearly and sincerely acknowledge the importance of whatever has triggered the aggression. Much violence results from the frustration that people feel when their own concerns are not being taken seriously.

2. Try to understand what the person is trying to achieve through being aggressive. If they want to dominate and take control, be passive and let them have control; if they want to escape, provide a way of allowing that. Think what their immediate needs are and try and satisfy them so that they do not have to use violence.

THE AFTERMATH OF A VIOLENT INCIDENT

It has been shown that violent incidents can have very long-term deleterious effects, and many victims could be defined as suffering from post-traumatic stress syndrome (DSM III, 1987). It is also known that intervention following the incident can reduce the number, intensity and longevity of these effects. Therefore, it is imperative that the psychological trauma of being involved in the incident is recognized both by the victim and those around them, and appropriate action should take place.

This action might take the form of counselling. Colin Rowett has done much work in this area, and has suggested that following such incidents workers will immediately experience fear, followed by surprise and then guilt (Rowett, 1986). Guilt is perhaps the most unexpected of these emotions, but also the most debilitating as it leads to self-doubt and lack of confidence.

In addition to counselling a person through these phases, it is also important to go through a systematic debriefing to find out what went wrong and how it can be prevented from happening again. As the victim is probably experiencing guilt and self-blame, it is tempting not to analyse what happened. However, if a thorough critical incident analysis is performed any deficits in training can be identified and filled.

CONCLUSION

It is hoped that this chapter has shown how understanding violent behaviour can help to prevent health professionals from placing themselves in unnecessary danger. There are further issues that have not been explored that have relevance to this area, such as 'How can we work therapeutically with people where control and fear are important issues for both client and therapist?'. However, it has been the aim of this chapter to raise the profile of violence in the workplace for those people working in the caring professions, and to give some basic, practical advice about how to avoid incidents.

REFERENCES

Argyle, M. (1984) *The Psychology of Interpersonal Behaviour*, 4th edn, Penguin, Harmondsworth.

Bandura, A. (1973) *Aggression: A social learning analysis*, Prentice Hall, New Jersey.

Breakwell, G. (1989) *Facing Physical Violence*, BPS/Routledge, Guildford.

Department of Health and Social Security (1988) *Violence to Staff: Report of the DHSS Advisory Committee on Violence to Staff*, HMSO, London.

Dollard, J., Doob, L., Miller, N., Mowrer, O. and Sears, R. (1939) *Frustration and Aggression*, Yale University Press, New Haven.

DSM III (1987) *Diagnostic and Statistical Manual of Mental Disorder*, 3rd edn, American Psychological Association, Washington.

Forgas, J.P. (1985) *Interpersonal Behaviour; The psychology of social interaction*, Pergamon Press, Oxford.

MacKay, C.J. (1987) *Violence to Staff in the Health Services*, HMSO, London.

McGurk, B.J., Davis, J.D. and Graham, J. (1981) Assaultive behaviour, personality and personal space, *Aggressive Behaviour*, **7**, 317–25.

Monahan, J. (1981) *Predicting Violent Behavior*, Sage, California.

Owens, G. and Ashcroft, B. (1985) *Violence: A guide for the caring professions*, Croom Helm, London.

Perkins, R., Hilton, M. and Pillay, H. (1991) *Clinical Psychologists' Experience of Violence at Work: Results of a national sample survey*. Available from R. Perkins, Clinical Psychology Dept, Springfield Hospital, London, SW17 7DJ.

Rowett, C. (1986) *Violence in Social Work*, Institute of Criminology Occasional Paper No. 14, Cambridge University.

Stout, K. and Thomas, S. (1991) Fear and dangerousness in shelter work with battered women, *Affilia: Journal of Women and Social Work*, **6**, no.2, 74–86.

5

Understanding, implementing and presenting counselling evaluation

Michael Barkham

OVERVIEW

The aim of this chapter is to provide practical guidelines to health professionals in addressing three questions: (1) Is counselling effective?; (2) How can health professionals evaluate their own practice?; and (3) How can health professionals best present data to managers in order to increase the resources allocated to them? In pursuit of these aims, a model of the health professional as a 'scientist-practitioner' is espoused in which each 'practitioner' (i.e. health professional) is also a 'scientist' (i.e. researcher) in that they can set up hypotheses, collect data, and evaluate particular aspects of their own interventions. Clearly, this evaluative aspect can take place at the moment-to-moment or session level of counselling with a client. Equally, it can take place at increasingly superordinate levels, such as the evaluation of change in an individual client or the effectiveness of the counselling practice. However, the aim of this chapter is not to present procedures for carrying out sophisticated studies of counselling outcome: such procedures have been well documented elsewhere (e.g. Shapiro, 1989). Rather, the purpose is to focus on how these procedures can be *applied* to everyday counselling settings and thereby integrated into a viable scientist-practitioner approach for health professionals.

IS COUNSELLING EFFECTIVE?

This question is the starting point for any debate concerning the effectiveness of individual health professionals and addresses the disciplines of counselling and psychotherapy, these terms being used interchangeably. The approach adopted in this chapter has been to look first at issues of methodology and then to provide an overview of the findings arising from the implementation of these methodologies and the various difficulties associated with them. More detailed accounts of the process and outcomes of individual therapy can be obtained elsewhere (e.g. Barkham, 1990).

Issues of methodology

To address the question of the general effectiveness of psychotherapy and counselling, three types of research design have been employed, each aimed at answering different parts of the outcome question. The first design is termed a *treatment vs. no-treatment* design in which the no-treatment condition acts as a control for extraneous factors (e.g. spontaneous remission). This design aims to address the question of whether therapy itself is more effective than no treatment at all. This question arose from Eysenck's (1952) critique of psychotherapy and led to a generation of research studies which aimed to 'justify' the practice of psychotherapy and counselling.

The second design is termed a *treatment vs. placebo* design in which a comparison is being made between an active treatment (i.e. counselling or psychotherapy) and what are generally termed 'common factors'. This design arises from the concern that the effective components in counselling and psychotherapy comprise factors which are common to all approaches (e.g. expectancy, hope, talking with someone, etc.).

The third design is termed a *comparative outcome* design and addresses the question of the differential effectiveness of two or more contrasting therapeutic orientations. This design aims to establish whether one form of counselling is more effective than another with the hope of identifying their specific effects.

The evidence from these three types of designs has been used in a recent approach termed *meta-analysis* which is a method for quantifying results from differing studies in order to arrive at an overall finding concerning the effectiveness of therapy. To achieve this, results from each study are standardized in the form of an effect size. An effect size is defined as the mean difference between treated and untreated groups at post-therapy divided by the standard deviation of the control group and enables comparisons to be made across studies. Hence, rather than simply saying that one treatment is better than another, research findings can now show how much better it is.

Overview of findings

The results from a series of meta-analytic studies led Lambert *et al.* (1986) to conclude that there 'is now little doubt ... that psychological treatments are, overall and in general, beneficial, although it remains equally true that not everyone benefits to a satisfactory degree' (p.158). Meta-analytic studies by Robinson *et al.* (1990) and Smith *et al.* (1980) reported findings from treatment vs. no-treatment control studies suggesting an effect size for therapy in the region of 0.84 and 0.85 of a standard deviation unit respectively. This is equivalent to the average treated client being better off than 80% of untreated clients. Comparing these effect size with those derived from clients with depression who were prescribed antidepressant medication, Andrews (Quality Assurance Project, 1983) found the effect sizes from antidepressant medication to range from 0.40 to 0.81. Accordingly, the effect size obtained in therapy studies is at least as good as those obtained from studies evaluating the effectiveness of psychotropic medication.

One of the main criticisms levelled at psychological interventions, and addressed by the treatment vs no-treatment design, is that improvement would have occurred in time without any form of specialized counselling. Eysenck (1952) pursued this argument suggesting that upwards of two-thirds of clients experiencing neurotic complaints improved without therapy within a two year period. More recent and considered research has suggested that Eysenck's figure was an overestimate and that the level is in the region of 43% (Lambert, 1986). It is important to appreciate that the fact of people reporting improvement without receiving psychological help does not argue against the effectiveness of counselling. Many psychological problems reflect periods of transitions in people's lives which ease with time. Similarly, some psychological problems (e.g. depression) have a cyclical nature and again may ease with time. However, this is not to say that psychological interventions might not enable the person to deal more effectively with problems at the time or that they will not have a prophylactic effect (i.e. enable the person to deal better with future problems). Overall, these findings have implications for the design of future studies. If studies have successively shown clients receiving treatment to improve more than those in control groups, then there are both scientific and ethical reasons for questioning the further utility of no-treatment control groups which are used for this purpose. Control groups may be appropriate in other situations.

Evidence from studies controlling for common factors, addressed by the placebo design, present a consistent but also challenging message for counselling. Results have continually found treated groups to show superior benefits to those clients receiving placebo interventions. For example, Smith *et al.* (1980) estimated the effect size for placebo controls to be 0.56, while Robinson *et al.* (1990) found only a non-significant effect size of 0.28 when the control condition was a placebo as against a waiting list control. Accordingly, while the evidence suggests a clear and consistent ordering of effects (i.e. clients receiving active treatments benefit more than those in placebo conditions who in turn benefit more than those in no-treatment conditions), it is clear that placebo treatments are by no means ineffective. This view is highlighted by the recent National Institute of Mental Health Collaborative Study of Depression (Elkin *et al.*, 1989). In this large-scale comparative study, while results indicated an ordering of effects in which the two active treatments (cognitive-behavioural and interpersonal therapy) were superior to a placebo condition, the findings were not statistically significant. Only with high severity clients did the active treatments perform significantly better than the placebo condition. This finding suggests that differences between active and placebo conditions may be small and only be apparent in more severe populations. A major point to consider is that psychotherapy studies adopting placebo controls are invariably looking for additive or incremental effects beyond those ascribed to the placebo. However, the finding that these *additive* effects are sometimes very slight does not argue that psychological therapies are ineffective.

However, there are considerable methodological problems with placebo designs when used to evaluate counselling and therapy. The placebo design derives from medical research in which any non-psychopharmacological effect of a drug can be evaluated by giving a placebo drug in which, by definition, the impact will be psychological. In addition, the provider can be blind to whether the drug is active or a placebo. Accordingly, specific and non-specific effects can be teased out. But these conditions cannot be applied to counselling. While placebo designs have served drug trials well, they are not sufficiently sophisticated to address psychological interventions. In addition, the nature of the intervention received by a placebo group should be a constituent part of the active treatment. Very often it is not and so, in effect, becomes a separate active treatment in its own right.

One procedure for lessening the methodological problems with placebo groups, while at the same time trying to establish what differences might exist between contrasting active treatments, has been the use of a comparative outcome design. What is particularly interesting here is that one might suppose that two very differing counselling approaches might lead to equally differing results. By contrast, the general view from comparative outcome studies is that the effects of counselling are broadly similar irrespective of the particular approach. This conundrum (i.e. differing therapies leading to broadly similar results) has been termed the *equivalence paradox* (Stiles *et al.* 1986). Accordingly, there is now an increasing trend focusing not so much on whether there are differences between the outcomes of therapies, but rather on addressing the question of what are the mechanisms by which a particular form of counselling or therapy works.

There are a number of implications arising from this situation. First, it may be the case that the equivalence of outcomes arises as a result of insufficiently sensitive research methodologies being used to identify differences between therapies – this is a methodological argument. There are many important issues here which are beyond the scope of this chapter but which are well summarized elsewhere (e.g. Shapiro, 1989). Second, it is possible that different therapies are broadly equivalent because although there are differences in technique, they have far more in common. This is the common factors argument and is a strong basis for arguing for the adoption of models of counselling which are characterized by eclectic or integrative approaches. Lambert (1986) estimated that the 30% of outcome variance which related to common factors was approximately twice that attributable to specific factors.

The factor most often identified as a common factor is the therapeutic relationship. Indeed, the therapeutic alliance can be viewed as the quintessential integrative variable because '... competent therapists of all persuasions are able to establish a positive emotional bond and a sense of mutual collaboration with receptive clients, and this...relationship carries most of the therapeutic weight' (Stiles *et al.*, 1986, p. 173). In a study comparing professional therapists with college professors, Strupp and Hadley (1979) determined the relative contribution of specific techniques versus common factors and concluded that positive changes were generally 'attributable to the healing effects of a benign human relationship' (p. 1135). In a classic American outcome study (Sloane *et al.*, 1975), a four month follow-up was carried out in which clients were asked to identify helpful components of therapy. The questionnaire included items on the therapeutic techniques as well as common factors. Clients, irrespective of the therapy they received, identified common factors as the most important. In a British outcome study, Stiles *et al.* (1988) found that while participating therapists rated sessions in relationship-oriented therapy as deeper than those in cognitive-behavioural therapy, clients did not differentiate between the two: for clients, therapy, regardless of theoretical orientation, was challenging and powerful (i.e. deep). Overall, both common and specific factors contribute to outcome, the role of both accounting for the broadly similar outcomes but at the same time recognizing that findings are not identical, carrying the implication that under certain conditions and with certain clients, some therapies may be more beneficial than others.

Before concluding this section, it is important to note the view, currently holding much favour, that it is erroneous to differentiate completely between the outcomes and processes (i.e. what happens in sessions) of counselling. There is increasing recognition that researchers need to look at counselling process and outcome together – as part of an integrated system. Consistent with this view, there is increasing interest in the 'events paradigm' (Elliott, 1983) which postulates that our understanding of counselling is best advanced by selecting for study those significant moments in therapy which lead to a critical shift in the client's state. Accordingly, the role of these significant moments (process) in achieving a change state within a session (i.e. mini-outcomes) is advanced and sets up an iterative process which is ongoing throughout counselling.

EVALUATING YOUR OWN PRACTICE.

The best way to go about evaluating counselling is first to decide what questions need to be answered. Accordingly, the nature and extent of the evaluation will be a function of for whom, or for what purpose, the questions are being asked. This section considers four main areas of evaluation: (a) service audit; (b) quality assurance; (c) effectiveness; and (d) cost-benefits, cost-efficiency and cost-effectiveness. More extended accounts of applied evaluation are available elsewhere (e.g. Parry, 1992; Rossi and Freeman, 1989).

Service audit

A service audit aims to find out who uses a service and how resources are allocated, and comprises systematic data collection and analysis. It therefore focuses on questions of service process and outcome. Primary candidates as variables within such an audit might include the following: age, gender, marital status, educational history, occupation, ethnic origin, and geographical location. This sociodemographic information can be informative in predicting future demands on the service and thereby help identify potential short-falls in service delivery. Beyond socio-economic information, it is then helpful to have some psychological information; for example, what is the range of problems with which people present? Having knowledge of this will signal specific needs in the service delivery, either in terms of particular presenting problems or particular client populations.

One advantage of the potential database for a service audit is that it will generally be available providing the basic information on clients has been logged. Accordingly, it is one form of evaluation which can, under most conditions, be retrieved albeit sometimes involving considerable work. A major reason why this data is more robust than most is that it is less prone to change: the demographic features of clients do not change in the space of a few months. By contrast, their psychological well-being can change considerably. In these situations, some type of sampling of clients' well-being has to take place prior to their attending for counselling. Although outcome data can be taken from counselling notes, the retrospective nature of this data means that it can be seriously flawed in many ways and is not generally advocated.

Quality assurance

Questions addressed by a quality assurance exercise focus on the process by which counselling is delivered and involves the setting and monitoring of standards for performance. Monitoring is achieved via a quality circle in which practitioners, rather than an external consultant, evaluate the quality of their service and devise and implement strategies for improving it. However, there is a considerable range in the standards which can be monitored. Well resourced practices might be able to monitor the quality of the counselling offered using audio tapes, peer supervision, and adherence manuals. Less well resourced practices may have to focus on more practical components of the service delivery: for example, time between initial referral and seeing a health professional.

Effectiveness

The issue of effectiveness, more than any other, is most synonymous with outcome. Questions of effectiveness include whether people receiving the service improve, and whether particular health professionals are more effective with some clients than others. The simplest form of evaluation is often referred to as a *pre- and post-counselling comparison* with the aim of showing that a change has occurred following the counselling intervention. However, difficulties arise in attributing change solely to the counselling intervention. Clearly, counselling has not been the only thing which has been taking place. Other major influences in the person's life could account for change. Addressing this problem would require a control group as described earlier in this chapter. In terms of what is applicable, we can help address the specific effectiveness of counselling by using each client as their own control through establishing a baseline for each client.

A baseline entails making a statement about the client's status across time prior to the counselling intervention. Health professionals need to know whether, in the time immediately prior to counselling, the client's problem is (a) stable, (b) deteriorating, or (c) improving. Because clients' moods can fluctuate, three assessment points are ideal, thereby enabling a U-shape or inverted U-shape curve to be plotted. With two pre-counselling assessment points, only a summary statement in which change (improvement or otherwise) is construed as linear can be made. However, the health professional can gauge whether improvement was occurring as a function of the client expecting to receive counselling. With only one pre-counselling assessment, the health professional has but a single snap-shot of the client's state and it is difficult to determine how stable this might be. However, this is the minimum requirement if the health professional is going to evaluate counselling interventions. Applying the same logic, assessments can be taken at various stages throughout counselling in order to inform the decision about when to terminate. In addition, administering assessments at follow-up, usually at three months or one year, also provides evidence for the impact of counselling.

These procedures can be applied to most clients in a counselling practice. However, an alternative, although not mutually exclusive, strategy is to employ a single case design in which the health professional adopts a more intensive study of a single client. This can be a mutually rewarding experience both for client and health professional. However, ground rules have to be explicit: for example, agreeing on whether the health professional has ongoing sight of the client's completed forms, in which case they become a means for the client communicating to the health professional, or whether the health professional only sees them at termination. There is a body of literature on single case methodology (e.g. Morley, 1989).

The use of self-report measures is a useful means of determining the level of effectiveness of counselling interventions, and each health professional will have their own preferences when it comes to deciding what measures to employ. However, if each health professional uses a measure unique to them, it makes it difficult, if not virtually impossible, to make comparisons between different practices and across geographical regions. The problem is balancing individuality with standardizing practice. A solution to this is to devise a 'core battery' which is universal but which allows individual health professionals to add measures either of particular interest to themselves or which they view as being important in the client's work.

A core battery can also be employed within a particular framework. The framework presented here comprises three levels: global, specific, and personal. The global level uses nomothetic measures because these, by definition, are the measures for which norms can be obtained. Accordingly, the core battery is derived from this level so that, ideally, all clients seen would complete the core battery which would enable counselling services to have a national overview of clients' presenting problems. Possible candidates for a core outcome battery might include short versions of the Symptom Checklist-90R (SCL-90R: Derogatis, 1983) and the Inventory of Interpersonal Problems (IIP: Horowitz *et al.*, 1988). Further information on these measures is presented in the Appendix on p. 81. Alternatively, the General Health Questionnaire (GHQ: Goldberg, 1978), of which there are versions of various lengths, might be suitable as a global measure. The second level (i.e. specific) might use nomothetic measures if available, but this level is the one which focuses on the particular issues of the client, for example, a particular phobia, an eating disorder, depression, etc.

In contrast to these two levels, the third level (i.e. personal) uses ideographic measures. Unlike nomothetic measures in which the client has no influence on the items, ideographic measures are characterized by the items they contain being devised by the client. In this way, each client can devise a procedure which is unique to their own experience while a level of standardization is achieved by there being a uniform scoring procedure. One easily devised format is the personal questionnaire method, originally devised by M.B. Shapiro (1961). For example, the most pressing issue for a client might be, in their own words, 'Worry over how I am dealing with my dementing mother'. This is a highly specific but very salient problem for the client's well-being. The point about these items is that they have personal meaning for the client because the client has devised them (e.g. Parry *et al.*, 1986).

In implementing any form of evaluation, there are some useful guidelines. First, be selective. Decide what question is being addressed and be focused – don't be tempted to do too much. It is far better to be able to arrive at a single clear finding about a specific issue than to arrive at inconclusive findings about a range of inter-related issues. Second, use more than one measure – change is a multifaceted process and no single measure will accurately summarize it. Using more than one measure enables a more realistic picture to be made of change, as in the hierarchy of measures detailed above (i.e. global, specific, and personal). Third, use multiple perspectives. The extent to which change is perceived to have taken place is influenced by whose perspective is taken. There is an increasing interest in sampling the perspective of, for example, the health professional, client, and perhaps a 'third party' (e.g. the client's partner or work colleague). Fourth, use multiple data points. The more data points there are, the more dependable the data becomes. In addition, greater numbers of data points enable a pattern of the change process to be plotted rather than a crude 'before and after' summary. And fifth, collect information on clients' life events during the course of therapy (some good and some not so good). Having a record of these events will enable the health professional (a) to monitor how the client is coping with issues which arise in everyday life, and (b) to provide data to help in addressing alternative explanations to the impact of therapy (i.e. that it was due to external effects).

Cost-benefit, cost-efficiency and cost-effectiveness

There is increasing pressure, both political and economic, to evaluate the cost of psychological interventions. A cost-benefit analysis aims to evaluate the costs and benefits of a programme solely in monetary terms. However, there are doubts about the validity of converting psychological outcomes into monetary units. A cost-efficiency study involves a comparison between two or more interventions in terms of the cost of achieving a desired and specified outcome. An example might be a comparison between the relative costs of two strategies for enabling a return to work for employees off work with stress. By contrast, in a cost-effectiveness study an outcome can be expressed either in more substantive or unspecified terms (e.g. psychological well-being) and aims to establish which intervention achieves the best therapeutic result in relation to the costs of implementing the intervention. The important point in a cost-effectiveness study is that only the costs of implementing the programme are expressed in monetary units. Ganster *et al.* (1982) carried out a study of stress management and concluded that it was generally effective but that they could not recommend its utilization due to the high cost of implementing and staffing the programme.

In addressing the need to take account of the effort and costs of carrying out an intervention, Newman and Howard (1986) advocated using the term 'therapeutic effort'. This concept comprises three components: dosage (i.e. the amount of counselling administered, usually in terms of number of sessions), restrictiveness (i.e. the constraints placed upon the client's life), and cumulative costs (total costs in terms of human and material resources). The authors present procedures for determining these various components. A simple example might involve a comparison between providing individual versus group counselling for 12 people. Evidence might show individual counselling to be more effective. However, the difference might not be sufficient to warrant the additional costs in terms of either the therapists involved or the waiting time demanded of the clients as a function of a therapist only being able to take on three clients for individual counselling at any one time. Another example is the question of weighing up the gains of providing an ongoing client with further counselling versus offering counselling to people waiting for a service. In light of the evidence of diminishing returns as the number of counselling sessions continue (Howard *et al.*, 1986), decisions have to be made as to how limited resources are best utilized to achieve the maximum therapeutic effect for people within the community.

HOW BEST TO PRESENT DATA TO MANAGERS

Health professionals may increasingly find themselves with the task of presenting data on their counselling practice to managers in a form which can support the need for maintaining existing resources and procuring additional ones. The aim of this section is to suggest various ways in which data can be presented to managers to serve these aims. Two points are worth noting. First, data should be contextual. By that is meant that a piece of data by itself can be used for a number of purposes depending on how you interpret it. In other words, the context in which the information is going to be used is paramount and data should be used in service of a specific argument and not in isolation. Second, it is helpful to differentiate between 'hard' and 'soft' data. Hard data is not only quantifiable, it is also objective and is therefore open to less questioning as to its validity and reliability. Examples of hard data include absenteeism rates, performance indicators, medication prescribed and any criterion-based indicator. Soft data can also be quantitative in nature but is less easy to verify from an independent source. Examples of soft data include all client self-report measures (qualitative and quantitative). One means of addressing this short-coming in self-report measures is to use third-party sources (e.g. work colleagues or partners). This is the principle of triangulation in which the aim is to show that reliance is not being placed solely on, for example, the client's perspective. This may be a challenge for counselling psychology as a discipline because much of its philosophy rests on 'valuing the person's perspective'.

Carrying out a cost-benefit exercise is a useful procedure. For example, it is one thing being able to show that providing a counselling service at a worksite leads to a decrease in the number of working days lost through 'sickness', but it is another to show that the cost of providing the service is outweighed by the returns in productivity for the company (i.e. that it is financially advantageous for the company to set up and maintain a counselling service). Similarly, if counselling allows couples to either 'mend or end' their relationships without resorting to expensive proceedings involving court costs, etc., then monies saved by the appropriate authority (e.g. DSS) might be usefully channelled directly to the counselling agency.

When costs are not of central importance, other procedures are needed to describe the benefits gained by clients from counselling. A procedure which is helpful is to be able to describe people after counselling as belonging to a different population as compared with before counselling. This is where data gathered prior to the commencement of counselling is so important. Data can be presented in at least two ways: as group data or individually. It can also be presented numerically or visually. For example, Barkham and Shapiro (1990) carried out a small pilot study of one form of counselling intervention with a sample of 12 clients who were assessed at six points in time using the Beck Depression Inventory (BDI: Beck *et al.*, 1961). A comparison between the first and fourth assessment showed a decrease in the mean BDI score for the group from 12.33 to 6.83, while at the sixth assessment the mean score was 4.27. A more powerful and informative way of presenting this data is to use graphs. Figure 5.1 plots the change across all the six assessment points with the BDI score marked on the right vertical axis. In addition, the left vertical axis marks the range of BDI scores using normative data for non-distressed populations obtained from a meta-analytic study by Nietzel *et al.* (1987). For non-distressed populations, they obtained a mean BDI score of

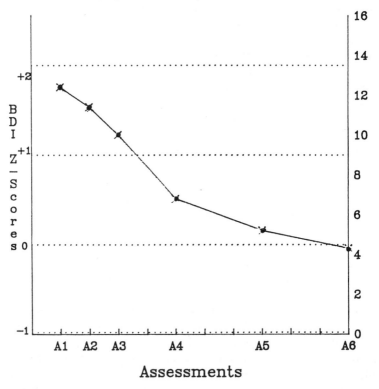

Figure 5.1 Effect sizes (z-scores) for pilot group compared with non-distressed norms.

4.54 (Sd = 4.46). The mean for the non-distressed population (i.e. 4.54) is marked as zero with each increasing standard deviation unit marked at increments of 4.46 BDI points. Figure 5.1 shows that at the first assessment the group mean approached 2 standard deviation units above the mean for a non-distressed population. It is common in psychology for people scoring more than 2 standard deviations above the norm to be identified as belonging to a different population. Figure 5.1 shows clearly that at the sixth assessment, the group mean for the 12 clients is just below the mean for the non-distressed population. Accordingly, it can be argued that these clients are best described as belonging to a non-distressed population.

Health professionals may also want to present data which identifies the progress of particular individual clients. In addi-

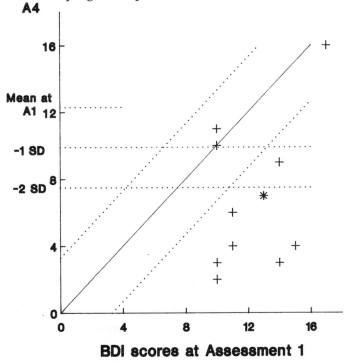

BDI scores at Assessment 1

* data for two clients

Figure 5.2 Assessing reliable and clinically significant change in a group of 12 clients

tion, they may be using a measure which does not have published or readily available norms. Figure 5.2 is drawn from the same data as above and presents the BDI scores of the 12 clients plotted between the first assessment (horizontal axis) and their fourth assessment (vertical axis). A client scoring the same at assessments one and four will be plotted on the diagonal (as indeed one is). The scores of clients who have improved (i.e. high at assessment one and low at assessment four) will be positioned towards the lower right-hand side of the graph. Indeed, anyone who has improved will be plotted to the right of the diagonal while anyone whose scores get worse will fall to the left of the diagonal. The diagonal dotted parallel lines mark the limits of measurement error for the instrument: details of this procedure can be obtained elsewhere (Jacobson and Truax, 1991). The horizontal dotted lines denote the 1 and 2 standard deviation boundaries calculated from the intake scores (mean 12.33; Sd = 2.35) and are used as in the previous example. The difference here is that we are taking the distressed scores as our starting point and working towards a boundary for the non-distressed population in which we hope their future scores will fall. Figure 5.2 shows eight of the 12 clients moving out of the distressed population by assessment four (i.e. beyond the 2 Sd boundary). This procedure enables the health professional to state that two-thirds of the clients met the criterion for membership of the normal population. Although this procedure may look complicated, it does not require a computer, although a pocket calculator might be useful. It can be built up and used as an ongoing means for evaluating change. However, as will be clear from this example, differing procedures lead to differing results.

Finally, it is important to remember that interventions with people within the normal population will show smaller effect sizes than those obtained in more clinical populations. In such instances, a different format should be used. One way to do this would be to use ideographic data. The appeal of this method is that it is more congruent with the philosophy of counselling psychology and yet provides quantitative data which is focused on the client's presenting difficulties. Another simple and yet effective way of presenting change data is in terms of some particular performance indicator or criterion-based measure. For example, with clients who have been off work, a relevant criterion could be 'return to (full-time) work'. In addition, clear statements about aspects of living which clients are now able to perform which they were unable to do previously are clear markers of improvement.

APPENDIX

In addition to general advice, further information can be obtained on the following:

1. Copies of the SCL-90R (and manual) and the IIP, together with their respective short versions.
2. The Service Evaluation Group acting under the auspices of the Society for Psychotherapy Research which publishes an occasional newsletter called Network. This provides a potential support system for work on evaluation;

from Dr Michael Barkham, MRC/ESRC SAPU, P O Box 604, Sheffield, S10 1FP.

REFERENCES

Barkham, M. (1990) Research in individual therapy, in W. Dryden (ed.) *Individual Therapy: A handbook*, 2nd edn, Open University Press, Milton Keynes.

Barkham, M. and Shapiro, D.A. (1990) Brief psychotherapeutic interventions for job-related distress: A pilot study of prescriptive and exploratory therapy, *Counselling Psychology Quarterly*, **3**, 133–47.

Beck, A.T., Ward, C.H., Mendelson, M., Mock, J. and Erbaugh, J. (1961) An inventory for measuring depression, *Archives of General Psychiatry*, **4**, 561–71.

Derogatis, L.R. (1983) *The SCL-90R: Administration, scoring and procedures – Manual II*, Clinical Psychometric Research, Towson, MD.

Elkin, I., Shea, M.T., Watkins, J.T., *et al* (1989) NIMH treatment of depression collaborative research program: General effectiveness of treatments, *Archives of General Psychiatry*, **46**, 971–82.

Elliott, R. (1983) Fitting process research to the practising psychotherapist, *Psychotherapy: Theory, Research and Practice*, **20**, 47–55.

Eysenck, H.J. (1952) The effects of psychotherapy: An evaluation, *Journal of Consulting Psychology*, **16**, 319–24.

Ganster, D.C., Mayes, B.T., Sime, W.E. and Tharp, G.D. (1982) Managing organizational stress: A field experiment, *Journal of Applied Psychology*, **67**, 533–42.

Goldberg, D. (1978) *Manual of the General Health Questionnaire*, NFER, Windsor.

Jacobson, N.S. and Truax, P. (1991) Clinical significance: A statistical approach to defining meaningful change in psychotherapy research, *Journal of Consulting and Clinical Psychology*, **59**, 12–19.

Horowitz, L.M., Rosenberg, S.E., Baer, B.A., Ureno, G. and Villasenor, V.S. (1988) Inventory of interpersonal problems: Psychometric properties and clinical applications, *Journal of Consulting and Clinical Psychology*, **56**, 885–92.

Howard, K.I., Kopta, S.M., Krause, M.S. and Orlinsky, D.E. (1986). The dose-response relationship in psychotherapy, *American Psychologist*, **41**, 159–64.

Lambert, M.J. (1986) Implications of psychotherapy outcome for eclectic psychotherapy, in J.C. Norcross (ed.) *Handbook of Eclectic Psychotherapy*, Brunner/Mazel, New York.

Lambert, M.J., Shapiro, D.A. and Bergin, A.E. (1986) The effectiveness of psychotherapy, in S.L. Garfield and A.E. Bergin (eds.) *Handbook of Psychotherapy and Behavior Change*, 3rd edn, Wiley and Sons, New York.

Morley, S. (1989) Single case research, in G. Parry and F.N. Watts (eds.) *Behavioural and Mental Health Research: A handbook of skills and methods*, Lawrence Erlbaum Associates, Hove.

Newman, F.L. and Howard, K.I. (1986) Therapeutic effort, treatment outcome, and national health policy, *American Psychologist*, **41**, 181–7.

Nietzel, M.T., Russell, R.L., Hemmings, K.A. and Gretter, M.L. (1987) Clinical significance of psychotherapy for unipolar depression: A meta-analytic approach to social comparison, *Journal of Consulting and Clinical Psychology*, **55**, 156–61.

Parry, G. (1992) Improving psychotherapy services: Applications of research, audit and evaluation, *British Journal of Clinical Psychology*, **31**, 3–19.

Parry, G., Shapiro, D.A. and Firth, J. (1986) The case of the anxious executive: A study from the research clinic, *British Journal of Medical Psychology*, **59**, 221–33.

Quality Assurance Project (1983) A treatment outline for depressive disorders, *Australian and New Zealand Journal of Psychiatry*, **17**, 129–46.

Robinson, L.A., Berman, J.S. and Neimeyer, R.A. (1990) Psychotherapy for the treatment of depression: A comprehensive review of controlled outcome research, *Psychological Bulletin*, **108**, 30–49.

Rossi, P.H. and Freeman, H.E. (1989) *Evaluation: A systematic approach*, 4th edn, Sage, Newbury Park, CA.

Shapiro, D.A. (1989) Outcome research, in G. Parry and F.N. Watts (eds.) *Behavioural and Mental Health Research: A handbook of skills and methods*, Lawrence Erlbaum Associates, Hove.

Shapiro, M.B. (1961) A method of measuring psychological changes specific to the individual psychiatric patient, *British Journal of Medical Psychology*, **34**, 151–5.

Sloane, R.B., Staples, F.R., Cristol, A.H., Yorkston, N.J. and Whipple, K. (1975) *Psychotherapy versus Behavior Therapy*, Harvard University Press, Cambridge, MA.

Smith, M.L., Glass, G.V. and Miller, T.I. (1980) *The Benefits of Psychotherapy*, Johns Hopkins University Press, Baltimore.

Stiles, W.B., Shapiro, D.A. and Elliott, R. (1986) 'Are all psychotherapies equivalent'? *American Psychologist*, **41**, 165–80.

Stiles, W.B., Shapiro, D.A. and Firth-Cozens, J.A. (1988) Do sessions of different treatments have different impacts? *Journal of Counselling Psychology*, **35**, 391–6.

Strupp, H.H. and Hadley, S.W. (1979) Specific vs. non-specific factors in psychotherapy: A controlled study of outcome. *Archives of General Psychiatry*, **36**, 1125–36.

Families

6

Having children, infertility and alternative family forms

Anne Woollett

Parenting is a major source of identity for adults. Becoming a parent is commonly viewed as a sign of adult status and as a significant transition during the life course. Children bring changes in what women and men do on a day-to-day basis, in their concerns and interests and how they relate to others. Relationships with children provide parents with emotional satisfaction, bring interest and variety into their parents' lives, and are a source of achievement and creativity. Parenting is often seen as adding to the meaning of life and ensuring personal development and continuity. At the same time parenting is costly and becoming a parent involves substantial adjustments for women and men. A general pattern of adjustment is often considered to characterize the transition women and men make as they become parents. However, parents' experiences, feelings and adjustments vary considerably and analysis of the factors associated with individual differences in adjustments suggest some of the problems and the benefits of parenting for women and men (Michaels and Goldberg, 1988; White and Woollett, 1992).

This chapter discusses a number of aspects of parenting. These are of relevance to health professionals whose work involves contact with women and men as they become or attempt to become parents. Health professionals who take care of women antenatally and at childbirth are aware of the range and variety of parents' feelings and adjustments. Sometimes these

may seem to be at variance with or raise questions about
strongly held ideas in medical circles about 'normal' or
'healthy' reactions and adjustments. Assumptions about parenting and family relations are also often questioned when
women and men experience reproductive difficulties. Assisted
reproduction, although it involves only a small proportion of
families, raises many difficult questions. Concern about the
moral and ethical issues involved in assisted reproduction led
to the setting up of the Warnock Committee which provided a
moral and legal framework for the treatment of infertility and
research on new reproductive technologies (Stanworth, 1987).

MOTHERING AND FATHERING

Parenting is in many respects similar for mothers and fathers,
but there are important differences in men and women's identities, experiences and activities as parents (Busfield, 1987).
Motherhood is a central aspect of women's identity, especially
when other outlets for achievement and creativity are limited.
But motherhood also has negative consequences as it restricts
women's opportunities to engage in other activities (Llewelyn
and Osborne, 1990). This happens in part because the circumstances of mothers' lives make it difficult for them to engage in
other activities, but stereotypes about women ensure that few
opportunities are available. Such stereotypes circumscribe the
lives of all women, whether they are mothers or not, irrespective of their children's age and hence the work involved in
caring for them, and women's social and financial circumstances
(Phoenix *et al.*, 1991). In contrast, fatherhood is less central to
men's lives and identities; men continue to view employment
as providing a major source of identity and fatherhood is not
expected to impinge significantly on their commitment to employment (Busfield, 1987).

Relations with children exist within the context of other
networks of relationships. For those in stable relationships,
these include most importantly those between parents. Parents'
relationships with their partners affect how well they adjust to
parenthood (Belsky *et al.*, 1984). The demands of a baby may be
experienced as emotional overload, as competition for a partner's
attention or as a shared activity and commitment. The responsibility of caring for a new baby may be stressful especially for

those who have difficulties with dependency relationships in general. The extent to which each partner acknowledges and respects the parenting skills of the other influences women's and men's confidence and satisfaction with parenting (Belsky *et al.*, 1984; Bronfenbrenner, 1986).

Parents' adjustments are also influenced by their own and the wider community's expectations of what it is to be a mother or a father. Fathers are now expected to be involved in the care of young children but discrepancies between what men do and what they and their partners consider appropriate are common and can be a source of dissatisfaction (Busfield, 1987). The support of the wider family also affects how well men and women make the adjustments parenting requires. Relationships with the parents' own families are often renegotiated as parents become grandparents and brothers and sisters become uncles and aunts. Women and men find they have more in common with their own parents once they are parents themselves.

SOCIAL CIRCUMSTANCES

Women and men become parents and bring up children in a variety of situations, some of which are considered more acceptable and desirable than others. It is expected, for example, that babies should be born to mothers married to or in a stable relationship with the baby's father. However, many mothers do not have the support of male partners. Single mothers are not a homogeneous group: their circumstances and experiences vary widely. Some bring up children on their own, and others live with and have the support of their own families. Women become single parents if their relationship with the child's father breaks up. For many women single parenthood is a short-lived phase which terminates as they enter into stable relationships (White and Woollett, 1992).

It is also considered that babies should be born when mothers are not too old nor too young. At present in the UK most children are born to mothers in their 20s and 30s, with comparatively few born to women under 20 or to women in their 40s. Motherhood is considered problematic for young women and has been linked to factors such as low infant birth weight, dependence on welfare benefits, poor mother-infant relations and poor educational outcomes for women and children.

However, recent evidence indicates that many young mothers and their children fare reasonably well and that any problems they experience are associated not with their youth so much as factors such as poverty, poor housing, unemployment and parity (young mothers are usually having first babies and for this reason are at greater risk of birth complications). Single or young women are assumed to have more negative attitudes to motherhood than women in their 20s and 30s or women in stable relationships. This may be the case for many women, but many younger and older women feel positively about motherhood and do not view themselves as disadvantaged (Phoenix *et al.*, 1991). In contrast we have less information about the factors associated with the reactions and adjustments of married women in their 20s and 30s.

The birth of a child changes the social circumstances of men's and women's lives. Commonly, women give up paid employment outside the home shortly before the birth of a first child. This is often associated with a sense of isolation, especially if women do not have friends or family living close by. In recent years, more women have begun to return to employment while their children are young and combine motherhood with employment. This often means a change from full-time to part-time employment as women try to find employment which fits around child care (Brannen and Moss, 1988).

Changes in family circumstances brought about by divorce and remarriage also have an impact. These are discussed in Chapters 7 and 8. Fathers' involvement in parenting is reduced with divorce but may increase later if they remarry and take care of stepchildren or children born into the new relationship. Children tend to stay with mothers when parents divorce so it is more common for children to live with stepfathers than with stepmothers. However, adjustments for stepmothers and children appear to be more difficult than is the case for stepfathers, suggesting that different dynamics underlie stepmothering and stepfathering (Smith, 1990) (see also Chapter 8).

For all parents, the support available from partners, families and friends is a major factor influencing their experiences. Social support takes a variety of forms and operates in different ways to help women and men cope with the changes parenting brings. Support may ease the material and financial pressures parents experience when mothers cease paid employment but want to purchase baby clothes and equipment. Support may consist of offering practical help and information. It may also take the form of baby-sitting to give parents 'childfree' time together. Support may operate at a more psychological level by helping parents to acknowledge their feelings and recognize any difficulties they are having. Parents can support each other and enhance one another's confidence by showing that they understand their partner's feelings and by their respect for one another's parenting skills (Wolkind and Zajieck, 1981; White and Woollett, 1992).

INDIVIDUAL DIFFERENCES

Reactions and adjustments to parenting vary widely over time and from individual to individual. Women's reactions are often linked to factors such as their personality or their relations with their mothers (Michaels and Goldberg, 1988). Women's adjustments may vary during pregnancy according to factors such as their physical symptoms and their reactions to discovering they are pregnant. Women who are pleased to be pregnant may begin to feel less positive if they experience severe symptoms in pregnancy or post-natally or their circumstances change, for example, if they become homeless or lose a close friend (Nicolson, 1986; Wolkind and Zajieck, 1981).

The medical management of pregnancy and childbirth affects women's feelings. Tests provide reassurance but they also create anxiety for which women need support from health professionals. Sometimes women resist thinking about their pregnancy as 'real' until they have the results of tests such as amniocentesis and until they accept that they really are pregnant they may find it difficult to act on advice from health professionals (Stanworth, 1987). Women's reactions to the medical management of childbirth also vary; while some women view procedures such as induction and fetal monitoring positively, others feel helpless and alienated from what they feel should be a good experience (Llewelyn and Osborne, 1990).

Although men often see themselves as being less actively involved in decisions about becoming a parent, most feel positive about their partner's pregnancy and feel that it has improved their relationship. Most fathers are now present at birth where they expect to provide practical and emotional support.

Fathers' presence is usually (but not always) welcomed by mothers as well as fathers and is often viewed as a prelude to their involvement in childcare, although there is no evidence that being present at birth necessarily increases fathers' later involvement (White and Woollett, 1992).

Parity (that is, whether a first or subsequent child) also influences parents' adjustments. The minority of studies which look beyond the initial transition to parenthood point to some differences in becoming a parent and parenting a second or third time. Parents of second and subsequent children already have experience of pregnancy and childbirth and usually feel more confident about their parenting skills. But a new baby creates extra work and increases the pressures on parents as they try to balance the needs of two or more children and later to manage sibling relationships to ensure that children get on well together (Phoenix *et al.*, 1991). The birth of a second child is often characterized as a difficult time for first children but there are also positive aspects as children play together and provide company for one another (Dunn, 1984).

Children's gender, health and personality also influence their parents' experiences. When their child is handicapped, for example, parents often find their own (and other people's) ideas about childcare are inappropriate for their child (Phoenix *et al.*, 1991; White and Woollett, 1992).

PROBLEMS IN BECOMING A PARENT

A significant number of men and women experience difficulty in becoming parents. Sometimes women cannot conceive because of problems with themselves or their male partners (Pfeffer and Woollett, 1983). Other women conceive easily but then find it difficult to maintain a pregnancy (miscarriage) or to deliver a live baby (stillbirth). Reproductive problems mean that people never become parents or do so only after a delay or after medical treatment. Sometimes people who cannot have their 'own' children become parents because they adopt children or become step-parents by caring for their partner's children from a previous relationship.

Not being able to become a parent is often experienced as loss, including loss of control of bodily functioning and of their lives. Childless men and women (but especially women) are seen in negative terms as deviating from generally accepted norms which emphasize the value of parenting. They have to come to terms both with their loss and subsequent grief and with the negative stereotypes associated with childlessness (Phoenix *et al.*, 1991). How men and women deal with reproductive problems depends in part on the cause, when one can be identified, and whether childlessness is a temporary state. When the problem lies with the man rather than the woman and persists for a long time, adjustments are more difficult. While some men and women accept their childlessness, others try to overcome it through adoption or medical treatment. The emotional reactions of women and men with reproductive problems may be difficult for health professionals to handle because they raise anxieties about their own fertility and parenting skills.

ALTERNATIVE FORMS OF FAMILY BUILDING

Adoption

Adoption is a traditional way of overcoming childlessness. Bringing up children they did not conceive or give birth to provides children for adoptive parents and parents for children who would otherwise have no family. In the past only non-handicapped babies were adopted but older children and handicapped children are now being adopted (Brodzinsky and Schechter, 1990; Tizard, 1977). When older children are adopted, they have experiences their parents do not share and parents may be anxious about whether they can form close relationships with their children. This anxiety may be reinforced by accounts of development which, in spite of the lack of evidence, stress the significance of early mother-child relationships for later development. Parents' concerns about children's background and parentage and about the reactions of others, including grandparents, to the adopted child may also add to their concerns.

Adoptive parents tend to be older than children's biological parents, they are more likely to be middle class and, because it is often a prerequisite for adoption, are more likely to be married or living in stable relationships. Because they have experienced problems in conceiving, adoptive parents' commitment to parenting may also differ. They will have had to consider parenting more seriously than parents who conceive easily but at the same time infertility investigations and the adoption process may have undermined their confidence.

The age at which children are adopted may have an impact on children's and parents' experiences of adoption. When children are adopted as babies their awareness of their adoption comes gradually and in the context of their adopted family. Children adopted at a later age have clearer understandings of what adoption entails and may have a history of disrupted relationships before they are adopted (Haimes and Timms, 1985; Tizard, 1977). Their awareness of the differences between themselves and other families may be increased if children come from different ethnic/cultural communities than their adoptive parents.

Assisted reproduction

A common response to infertility is to seek medical treatment. Three forms of assisted reproduction or reproductive technologies are discussed here.

Artificial insemination by donor (AID). With AID, sperm from a donor are used to enable the partner of an infertile man to conceive. The woman carries and gives birth to the child which the couple care for and bring up as their own. Apart from the conception, there are few practical ways in which being the mother of an AID child is different from that of mothering a child conceived more traditionally. An AID child has her/his mother's but not father's genes. It is often considered that the lack of genetic links between father and child reduces fathers' commitment to the child but fathers can (and usually do) show their commitment by their involvement in the pregnancy or by participating in the child's upbringing (Humphrey and Humphrey, 1988; Stanworth, 1987).

The psychological significance for parents and children of being conceived through AID has not been investigated. The major impact of AID may result from parents' concern about differences between their own children and those conceived conventionally and about children's reactions to finding out about their conception.

In vitro fertilization (IVF) allows some women to conceive children using their own or donated eggs. It involves obtaining ova (eggs) from the woman, mixing them with her partner's sperm (conception) and, if the fertilized eggs begin to divide, placing them in the woman's uterus (implantation). A baby born as a result of IVF carries the mother's and her partner's genes (or, with donated eggs, her partner's but not the woman's genes). Because IVF has a low success rate, it is common to implant more than one fertilized egg to improve the chances of establishing a pregnancy. This increases the effectiveness of IVF, but also makes a multiple pregnancy more likely.

Twins and other multiples are associated with complications of pregnancy and birth, higher perinatal mortality rates, and difficulties and costs of childcare (Botting *et al.*, 1990). As with AID, it is not clear what the effects of a technological and stressful means of conception might be for parents or on parents' relationship with the child (Stanworth, 1987).

Surrogacy has emerged recently as another 'alternative' form of family building. Here one woman (surrogate mother) contracts to carry and give birth to a child for another (receiving mother) who subsequently brings up the child. In some respects surrogacy is similar to adoption except that the agreement between the surrogate and receiving mother is made prior to the child's conception rather than after the child's birth. Usually the child shares some of the receiving parents' genes but is carried by and born to another woman (Stanworth, 1987).

These techniques raise difficult practical and moral questions for would-be parents and for health professionals about how they feel about intervening in reproductive processes. Health professionals also have to consider the resource implications of assisted reproduction. When resources are scarce, difficult decisions have to be made about who is offered treatment and who is not.

As with other less dramatic infertility investigations, little is known about the ways in which people cope with infertility treatment and, if successful, with pregnancy, birth and bringing up children. Some parents argue that children conceived after investigations are 'special' and this influences how they feel about them and bring them up. However, others argue that once they become parents, reproductive difficulties fade into insignificance in the day-to-day activities of childcare (Pfeffer and Woollett, 1983).

SOME ISSUES RAISED ABOUT PARENTING

The number of families created by adoption and these 'medical' forms of family building is relatively small. In the UK about 1000 babies and 4000 older children were adopted in 1988, about 1200 were born as a result of IVF, and probably twice as many conceived through AID compared with a total of about 780,000 births (Humphrey and Humphrey, 1988). They do, however, indicate some of the issues around parenting which are important to all parents and health professionals working with parents.

Parents often feel that children provide a sense of continuity and commitment to the future which is articulated in terms of genetic links with children but also through joint activities and interests with the next generation. In conventional families these social and biological aspects of parenting overlap. With 'alternative' forms of family building, the genetic link between parents and children may be partially or completely broken, although the social relationships are maintained. With AID, IVF and often with surrogacy (as with step-parenting) there are genetic links between parents and children. Children conceived through AID have their mother's but not their father's genes. With adoption the parent-child relationship is built entirely on the caring and commitment of parents and children (Humphrey and Humphrey, 1988; Schaffer, 1986).

Another issue which is sometimes articulated relates to children as resulting from or being an expression of parents' sexual relationship. With IVF a couple may have 'their' child, but (as with AID and surrogacy) the process by which the ova and sperm are brought together is clinical and lacking intimacy. On the other hand, many parents argue that going through such treatments (as with adoption procedures) brings them a closeness which compensates for the clinical way in which their children were conceived (Pfeffer and Woollett, 1983). Such concerns relate only to the conception and/or birth of their child. Once they become parents men and women are engaged, like other parents, in bringing up children and are accepted as parents by others.

Often parents fear the reactions of others to their infertility or to the child's origins and so prefer to remain silent about how their families have been formed. When parents adopt an older child or a child from a different ethnic community, the differences between their family and conventional families cannot be hidden but in other cases differences are less obvious and families can, if they wish, keep their secret and 'pass' as conventional families. Keeping silent helps families to maintain the appearance of conventionality but maintaining secrets can be costly. Energy goes into hiding rather than dealing with issues and people never have the opportunity to obtain support from others. It is rare for a secret to be really hidden so there is always the risk that children will be told by others (Haimes and Timms, 1985; Humphrey and Humphrey, 1988). With adoption it is current policy to tell children that they are adopted and to give them information about their biological parents. But those who become parents through the use of assisted reproduction are advised by health professionals to remain silent and indeed often parents have little information to give a child about a sperm or egg donor. The need for such secrecy is questioned by some parents and health professionals.

CONCLUSION

Parenting provides many men and women with an important aspect of identity and emotional satisfaction but as they become parents and bring up children, they make substantial and sometimes difficult adjustments. The nature of these adjustments and parents' experiences of parenthood are influenced by a variety of factors including their gender, their relationship with their partner and the characteristics of children. In this context the impact of the attitudes of health professionals and the support they can provide also need to be considered. Parenting has an impact on and is influenced by events in other areas of people's lives such as the wider family, employment and other extra-familial commitments (Bronfenbrenner, 1986).

A number of alternative ways of creating families used by those with fertility problems have been discussed. Examination of these family forms points to issues of importance for parents and children in such families and for health professionals involved with such families. But they also throw light on what

parenting means for all men and women and for the wider
society. Alternative forms of family creation usually involve a
separation of biological and social aspects of parenting and
hence raise questions about the relative significance of each for
parents' relationship and commitment to their children. Also,
because these forms of family creation involve medical and/or
adoption professionals, they raise difficult issues for health
professionals. They also bring into the public arena areas of life
which are usually considered to be largely private and by doing
so indicate the ways in which family building is of public
concern and subject to public control (Schaffer, 1986).

REFERENCES

Belsky, J., Robins, E. and Gamble, W. (1984) The determinants of paren-
tal competence: towards a contextual theory, in M. Lewis (ed.) *Beyond the Dyad*, Plenum Press, New York.
Botting, B.J., Macfarlane, A.J. and Price, F.V. (1990) *Three, Four and More:
A study of triplet and higher order births*, HMSO, London.
Brannen, J. and Moss, P. (1988) *New Mothers and Work*, Unwin Paper-
backs, London.
Brodzinsky, D.M. and Schechter, M.D. (eds.) (1990) *Psychology of Adop-
tion*, Oxford University Press, Oxford.
Bronfenbrenner, U. (1986) Ecology of the family as a context for human
development: research perspectives, *Developmental Psychology*, **22**, 723–42.
Busfield, J. (1987) Parenting and parenthood, in G. Cohen (ed.) *Social
Change and the Life Course*, Tavistock, London.
Dunn, J. (1984) *Sisters and Brothers*, Fontana, London.
Haimes, E. and Timms, N. (1985) *Adoption, Identity and Social Policy: The
search for distant relatives*, Gower, Aldershot.
Humphrey, M. and Humphrey, H. (1988) *Families with a Difference –
Varieties of surrogate parenthood*, Routledge, London.
Llewelyn, S. and Osborne, K. (1990) *Women's Lives,*. Routledge, London.
Michaels, G.Y. and Goldberg, W.A. (1988) *Transition to Parenthood: The-
ory and research*, Cambridge University Press, Cambridge.
Nicolson, P. (1986) Developing a feminist approach to depression fol-
lowing childbirth, in S. Wilkinson (ed.) *Feminist Social Psychology*,
Open University Press, Milton Keynes.
Pfeffer, N. and Woollett, A. (1983) *The Experience of Infertility*, Virago,
London.
Phoenix, A., Woollett, A. and Lloyd, E. (eds.) (1991) *Motherhood: Mean-
ings, practices and ideologies*, Sage, London.
Schaffer, H.R. (1986) Child psychology: the future, *Journal of Child
Psychology and Psychiatry*, **27**, 761–79.
Smith, D. (1990) *Step-mothering*, Harvester Wheatsheaf, Hemel Hemp-
stead.

Stanworth, M. (1987) *Reproductive Technologies; Gender, motherhood and medicine*, Polity Press, Oxford.
Tizard, B. (1977) *Adoption: A second chance*, Open Books, London.
White, D. and Woollett, A. (1992) *Families: A context for development*, Falmer, Basingstoke.
Wolkind, S. and Zajieck, E. (1981) *Pregnancy: A psychological and social study*, Academic Press, London.

7

Family break-up and divorce: balancing the costs and benefits

David White

It is estimated that 30% of children with married parents will experience family break-up in Britain by the year 2000 and rather more of children with non-married parents (Wicks and Keirnan, 1990). Estimates for the USA put the figures much higher at over 50% (e.g. Hofferth, 1985). Professionals may become involved with these families at various points, including: marriage counselling before a decision to part has been made; conciliation during the period of the break-up, including negotiations about custody and visitation arrangements; assisting and advising parents on childcare; treating cases of stress-induced illness or depression among parents and children; intervening when children are seen to be out of control, or when they are suspected of being abused or neglected; and coping with emotional and health problems of older children such as substance abuse or unwanted pregnancies.

In their training most professionals are introduced to psychological theories stressing the importance of continuing intimate relationships in ensuring physical and psychological well-being. Theories of child development stress the importance of enduring attachments to both parents and theories in adult health psychology emphasize the importance of satisfying relationships with the partner and partner support. With family break-up there is discontinuity of intimate relationships; children's attachments to parents become modified and the nature of adult relationships changes. On the surface those psychological theories suggest that family break-up will have adverse long term effects on all family members, but especially on the development of children. This chapter examines this proposition by summarizing the available evidence about the effects of break-up on the family and then attempts to weigh up the costs and benefits of this action.

EFFECTS OF BREAK-UP ON THE FAMILY

Most of the evidence about the effects of family break-up comes from comparisons of families broken by the departure of a parent with matched intact two-parent families. From this it is clear that the transitions following separation or divorce are highly stressful for all the family (Gorell Barnes, 1991). Family break-up leads to a number of changes in the lives of all family members: they cope to varying extents with their sense of personal rejection; adjust to new routines in their lives; frequently experience financial hardship; and many experience environmental change, no longer living in the same physical location surrounded by the same familiar belongings. Any of these changes could have an impact on children and their parents and could contribute to any problems that follow in the wake of family break-up.

Family adjustments over time

The year following family break-up is a period when few family members function well. Most men and women feel depressed, incompetent, angry and rejected and even after one year many regret the separation. For both partners the development of a new intimate relationship helps them to restore their confidence and come to value themselves again. For many custodial parents this first year of bringing up children without the former partner is especially hard. Many are socially isolated, receive little support with parenting, work long hours, experience stressful life changes and their lives become more restricted to interactions with or about children. For their part, children respond negatively to the changes in their lives during this early period, although this is affected in part by their age and gender.

Children of all ages show initial depression, unhappiness and anxiety, they become inattentive to others, not entering into interactions with friends and family as readily as before, they engage in less cooperative play, play less overall and are more likely at this time to express themselves aggressively. Consequently, immediately following family break-up children tend to become socially isolated, and for boys this frequently continues, as former friends continue to shun them, even when later they attempt to reintegrate themselves. Younger boys and girls also display more clinging, whining, complaining and aggression as well as more oppositional behaviours, refusing to do things they are asked to do. In the year following separation children commonly fear abandonment by the custodial parent and ridicule from friends and peers; at this time self-blame is common too. In the second year these fears decrease. After about a year girls typically show quite a marked improvement in their behaviour and in the face that they present to the world, but for boys the apparent improvement is much less. Even after two years they are more socially isolated, less cooperative and more obviously unhappy (Hetherington, 1988).

In the longer term the effects of family break-up can be seen in boys' and girls' poor impulse control, aggressiveness, noncompliance and under-achievement. On average the under-achievement of children is quite modest when account is taken of their pre-separation social backgrounds. However, these averages conceal some individuals who are faring badly. Age and gender of children are important here and are discussed in the next two sections.

Age of children

Initially, all children, whatever their age, feel unhappy and insecure after the break-up. However, infants and preschool children tend to be the most frightened, confused and sad age group, often worrying about their own contribution to their parent's departure. They reveal the greatest problems in the first year or two. Older, school aged children show less sign of distress although their behaviour and their schoolwork deteriorate, especially in the case of boys. They begin to be able to understand that their parents might be incapable of living together and they can see the benefits of reduction in family conflict. Adolescents are most likely to see positive outcomes of the divorce, to see it as triggering their own increased sense of self-reliance and responsibility and to see their parents undergoing positive personality changes (Kurdek, 1986).

Although in the short term younger children are more adversely affected than older, this position changes with the passage of time. Ten years after the separation younger children rarely remember their pre-separation lives, they perceive their relationship with their parent as being good and are optimistic about their own futures. They remain confident about marriage, expecting to get married themselves and their marriages to last. In contrast, older children look back on the break-up as a time of great personal unhappiness; they see their idealized childhood as having been snatched away from them. This group see the divorce as having had a powerful influence on their lives. At this time there is still a yearning for the family to be reunited and this feeling is stronger the older the child at the time of the break-up (Wallerstein *et al.*, 1988).

Sex of children

In the short term girls appear to cope with family break-up better than boys, although this may occur because boys and girls express their distress in different ways with boys' expressions of distress being more visible than girls' and harder to ignore. Following the break-up boys demonstrate more externalizing behaviours such as aggressiveness, poor attention, delinquency and antisocial problem behaviours. In contrast, girls' behaviours may not impinge so much on their caretakers and may not be recognized therefore as distress; girls are more likely to display internalizing behaviours such as anxiety, withdrawal and depression. Although some of the apparent difference in the reactions of the sexes can be explained by different expressions of distress, boys do indeed show a more adverse reaction to their parents' break-up, and especially when living with their mother as the lone parent (Zaslow, 1989).

Following break-up both sons and daughters are allowed more responsibility and independence than children of the same age from intact families. As part of this parents monitor their children less, being less likely to know where they are or who they are with, and they are more likely to leave their children alone and unsupervised in the home. On this regime girls feel they are growing up faster than they would have done had the family stayed together and they report having a satisfying relationship with their parent. Boys report behaving aggressively and being non-compliant to parental requests and frequently engaging in antisocial acts: parents are frequently unaware of these.

One reason boys have more adverse reactions than girls is that they are less effective in soliciting help and support from others and in particular they are poor at disclosing their feelings and their anxieties. Sharing problems and worries usually helps individuals to find solutions and diminishes the experience of stress. Professionals can play an important part in encouraging self-disclosure and in training children to utilize the help that is usually available. Many adults as well as children do not know how to express their needs to others and elicit help. Training in these skills can be a highly effective intervention.

In the longer term the effects of family break-up on girls become more apparent. Adolescent girls from broken homes are more rebellious, more involved in precocious sexual activity, have a greater involvement in alcohol and drugs, show higher rates of depression and experience more difficulty in their heterosexual relations than do girls from intact homes (Hetherington, 1988). Even in adulthood a significant minority of women are very fearful of making commitments to others, fearing betrayal, although a close relationship with a sibling appears to offer reassurance that other relationships can be successful too. In the long term women brought up as children in homes broken by either the death of a parent or family break-up describe their childhoods as less happy than do women from intact homes and as mothers they are less warm and demonstrative in their interactions with their own children (Wadsworth, 1985).

Following family break-up more than 80% of children remain with their mothers, although this is affected by the age and sex of children. Fathers have custody of boys, and especially adolescent boys, more frequently than girls and they are least likely to have custody of girls under the age of two years. Father custody is less common, but girls fare worse in these cases, as they do when they are in a stepfather family (Zaslow, 1989). A study of British women suggests that the loss of the mother is frequently associated with inadequate parental care which in the long term can have adverse effects for women, resulting in an increased incidence of clinical depression. The loss of the mother only becomes important when women experience other adverse life events. Women without a mother are less likely to have developed the resources that will allow them to cope and in particular their evaluation of themselves (self-esteem) is lowered. Moreover, motherless women are more likely to experience certain adverse life events such as premarital pregnancy and the break-up of their own intimate relationships than are women with available mothers (Bifulco *et al.*, 1987). Children cope best with family break-up when they are cared for by a custodial parent of the same sex as themselves, revealing fewer behavioural problems.

Maintaining routines

One cost of break-up for many separating families is the lowering of family income, resulting in real and enduring financial hardship for the custodial parent and children. Studies have shown that family break-up has a twofold impact on the development of children: a direct effect of the loss of a parent and the loss of the family identity and an indirect impact through lowered family income and an accompanying change in family lifestyle and routines. In those cases where family income remains 'good enough', children show much less distress at family break-up. In these cases custodial parents are better at maintaining pre-separation routines and show greater tolerance of disruptions in their children's behaviour. Professional help in gaining available state benefits or maintenance payments will consequently not only assist the family materially, but will limit their members' psychological distress.

In the first year following the break-up average custodial parents are poor at maintaining pre-separation routines consistently for themselves and their children. The custodial parent is less likely to eat meals with their children than before, to read to them or to play with them, to get them to school and to appointments on time, and is more erratic in getting them to bed. These disruptions to routines are most likely to occur when the custodial parent is pre-occupied about money worries or with their own adjustment problems (Hetherington, 1988).

Consistency of parenting

Especially in the short term, family break-up can result in the custodial parent displaying less consistent and sensitive parenting because of anxieties about money and about themselves. In the two years following family break-up custodial parents make few maturity demands of their children and are inconsistent in their disciplining. In the short term there are fewer maturity demands because it is easier to do things for the child rather than nagging the child to complete the task properly. Inconsistent disciplining takes the form of restrictive rules that are poorly enforced. Both compliance and non-compliance are frequently ignored and so children do not receive clear feedback about the appropriateness of their behaviour.

Deterioration in the effectiveness of parenting can be increased by parental depression and tiredness which leads to a lowered tolerance of child behaviours. In part this occurs because depressed parents only attend to the child when forced to by inappropriate behaviours that in fact have a low frequency, but because of selective attention are seen as being highly representative of the child's behaviour. The child is seen as deviant and so parents increase their attempts at authoritarian control. In turn this leads to more conflict between the two, the parent perceiving the child as still more difficult and adopting increasingly ineffective child management strategies. This adds to the burden placed on the child by the loss of the non-custodial parent.

Some of the distress of children at family break-up is exacerbated by the custodial parent's parenting behaviours. Immediately after the separation children's overt behaviour changes little, but their behaviour quickly deteriorates unless their parent displays sensitive and consistent parenting, providing a predictable environment with clearly defined and enforced rules. The less sensitive and predictable the parent's behaviour, the more oppositional, non-compliant and aggressive behaviours children exhibit (Brody and Forehand, 1988).

Difficulties in parent–child relationships may persist,

especially with boys. Even six years after the break-up mother/boy relationships can be problematic. Mothers spend less time with their sons than their daughters and report feeling less rapport with them and less close to them. Mothers are poor at controlling their sons, requests are frequently ignored and when this happens mothers tend not to pursue the request, although their interactions with sons consist of a lot of complaints and nagging. In interacting with sons, mothers are more likely to get involved in angry and lengthy exchanges. In contrast, mothers' feelings for girls are more positive, they feel closer to them and more in tune with daughters. Linked to this, mothers express more affection for daughters (Hetherington, 1988).

Children and adults show the best adjustments when their lives are predictable and stable. Encouraging parents to adopt regular routines and to show consistency in their parenting will benefit the whole family. To achieve this parents need to be encouraged to monitor their own and their children's behaviour more closely, so that they become more aware of the realities of what is happening in the family. With increased awareness, parents are in a position to modify family routines and improve their parenting. Other adults can be especially helpful in providing an alternative perspective on the behaviour and emotional state of children, and in providing feedback to parents about the appropriateness of their parenting. Helping parents utilize the support that friends and family can provide can be a valuable tool in improving the emotional and physical health of the entire family.

BALANCING THE COSTS AND BENEFITS

From the above summary it is clear that following family break-up some family members function poorly and may continue to do so for long periods. On the basis of this type of evidence the belief has developed in some quarters that children are best served by life in two-parent families even when the relationship between the parents is poor. However, this interpretation of the data may not be justified. The evidence does not of itself provide much of an insight into the relative costs/benefits of continued intact family life compared to family break-up.

Misleading evidence?

One area in particular where the evidence may be misleading is when looking for the long term effects of family break-up. Some of the British data reports on the adjustments of children 20 or more years on. For instance, Wadsworth and Maclean (1986) report that the lowered educational attainment of children frequently results in long term depressed socio-economic status, especially for men. These studies tend to produce a very negative view of the long term effects of family break-up, with adverse consequences continuing into children's adult lives, affecting their own parenting skills, their happiness, and their material and emotional well-being. They probably reflect accurately the experiences of children whose families broke up in the 1950s and 1960s. However they may or may not reflect the future experiences of children whose families break-up in the 1990s and beyond. It cannot be assumed automatically that recently separated families will become in time like earlier separated families. They may cope better or they may cope worse. Over the years the incidence of family break-up has changed dramatically, as have attitudes and social supports available to families in transition. These changes may mean that the recently separated will function differently from their longer separated counterparts.

A second feature of the evidence summarized earlier is that virtually all of it looks at the adjustments of family members post-separation; there is no information about how the family were coping pre-separation, or how families who remain together in disharmony cope. Although there are problems post-separation these may or may not be greater than those experienced prior to the break-up or in some intact families. For example, following divorce, children frequently report continuing unhappiness and dissatisfaction with life which they blame on the divorce. However, in evaluating these self-reports it is necessary to consider too how children who live in conflict or who suffer abuse report on their lives; only then can a picture of the effects of family break-up be constructed and a judgement made whether or not they are any less happy than their counterparts whose parents did not separate. Young adults who are unhappy look for an explanation of that unhappiness. In the case of children from broken homes the family break-up provides an explanation for their unhappiness.

Children from intact homes have to find alternative explanations if they feel unhappy and dissatisfied with their lives.

There are alternative forms of evidence which include more comparative data from which to judge the relative costs and benefits of both family break-up and continued life in disharmonious families. These studies point to the damage that family conflict can produce.

Family conflict

Family break-up is usually preceded by a build-up in tensions, with increased arguments and conflict in the home. Tension in the family is distressing for all family members and can have long term consequences on the adjustments of children of all ages. Anger and fighting in the home, whether it is physical or verbal, is upsetting for even very young children who feel less happy and secure because they are exposed to disagreements. Moreover, the more frequently conflicts occur the greater the distress shown by children. Even children of one and two years may attempt to defuse family conflicts by trying to create distractions or by mediating and trying to reconcile the arguing parties. Girls show distress to witnessed conflict to a more marked degree than do boys. Parental conflict is associated with conduct disorders and emotional difficulties in children and adolescents, including aggressive and delinquent behaviour, and boys seem more adversely affected than girls (Cummings *et al.*, 1985).

Indirectly, conflict can have an impact on children because it leads the conflicting participants to be less sensitive in their dealings with the rest of the family; they become pre-occupied with their own problems and needs and so fail to respond to the problems and needs of others. Family break-up can lead to less competent parenting, but so too can family conflict. Fathers' parenting is more affected by conflict and a deterioration in their relationship with their partner, but both parents show the same trend. Even without any open hostility the deterioration in the parental relationship will affect all family members. When there is conflict in the home, parenting becomes more distant and control more lax; it may also become more punitive, leading to children displaying the more negative internalizing and externalizing behaviours also associated with family break-up. Children are more adversely affected by poor parenting from mothers than fathers, reflecting the relative amounts of time that children spend with their mothers and fathers. However, fathers can contribute to child behavioural problems when they are irritable and frequently argue with their children.

Boys are more susceptible to parental disharmony than girls. Parents may terminate arguments quicker when with girls because girls show their distress to family conflict in a more pronounced manner than do boys. Additionally, boys are in general more demanding of attention and require more direct control than girls. Under normal circumstances parents seem able to cope with the extra demands of boys and perceive them in a positive light; however when parents are under stress, as they are when they are experiencing conflict, they become irritated by these demands and perceive them in a more negative light and respond less sensitively to the demands of sons. Daughters make relatively light demands and so those demands continue to be met in a sensitive way (Fauber *et al.*, 1990; Holden and Ritchie, 1991).

The impact of conflict on children is minimized if conflicts are resolved by a compromise being reached between the parents. In these cases children are better adjusted, exhibit more pro-social behaviours and have higher self-esteem. In contrast if conflicts are resolved by one parent verbally attacking the other, children show lower self-esteem and engage in more aggressive behaviours and fewer pro-social behaviours (Camera and Resnick, 1988).

Removing children from conflict

Family break-up is damaging to children, but so too is conflict. The decision about which family form best serves the interests of children is not clearcut. There are costs and benefits associated with either action. Children are capable of loving the most unlovely parents even when those parents abuse them; separation from those parents represents a loss of a known and predictable element in their lives. Despite this most of the evidence points to the advantages of removing children from conflict; it is the conflict that individuals experience that leads to some of the longer term effects of family break-up.

One valuable source of information in this respect are large scale household surveys (e.g. Furstenberg, 1988). In these studies, data is collected from a large number of families at one time point. Detailed information is gathered about the living arrangements of each family as well as information from health records, school records and so on. In this way a snapshot is taken of each family at one point in time. Because a large number of families are included, all types of family configurations will be sampled: some will be contented two-parent families, others discontented two-parent families, others recently separated one-parent families, others longer separated one-parent families. The different family forms can then be compared to see how the parents and children are coping in each family configuration. They find that children from conflict-ridden homes, whether broken or intact, are less well adjusted than children from conflict-free homes. Girls from conflict-free divorce are indistinguishable from girls of conflict-free marriages, although boys are adversely affected even when the divorce is conflict-free, but not as badly as they are by conflict in marriage.

Because of deteriorating family relationships prior to the break-up it is likely that children will already be suffering adverse consequences, but these accelerate as the break-up occurs. Longitudinal studies confirm that this happens. In these studies a large number of families are studied for several years; during this period some of them experience family break-up. In these cases it is possible to examine the effects of break-up and compare them to adjustments prior to the break-up (e.g. Doherty and Needle, 1991). As much as 11 years prior to break-up boys reveal the adverse behaviour typically revealed by boys immediately after divorce; in particular they show poor impulse control, high aggression and high activity levels. The effects are stronger the greater the marital conflict. Girls, and especially adolescent girls, also show the ill effects of parental conflict prior to family break-up. Pre-separation conflict has an adverse effect on children, but the family break-up has a further impact on boys who show increased substance misuse and a deterioration in their psychological well-being, including unhappiness, dissatisfaction with life and depression. In contrast, the psychological well-being of girls is not further eroded by the break-up.

There are advantages to removing children from conflict-ridden relationships; when they are removed from conflict they show rapid improvements. Unfortunately, family break-up does not necessarily lead to a reduction in family conflict and it may even escalate following the break-up. Following the break-up children may be exposed more directly to any conflict as parents use the children as sounding boards for their angers and frustrations with the late partner. The more conflict that they encounter the harder it is to cope. In general conflict diminishes after the first year of separation. Another reason why conflict may continue is that conflict between parents may be replaced by conflict between a parent and child or between parent and a step-parent.

The benefits to all family members of reducing their experience of conflict are clear, and it is important to attempt to reduce conflict during and after the break-up. Counselling directed at the diminishing of conflict and training in conflict resolution are important intervention strategies to be utilized during and after family break-up.

Although the family can be a very public place it is also a place where secrets can be maintained surprisingly well and children are often totally unprepared for the end of their parents' relationship, either because the parents have been good at concealing conflict and unhappiness from their children or because the children have chosen to turn a blind eye to the evidence of what has been happening.

SUMMARY AND CONCLUSIONS

Family break-up is frequently distressing, especially in the short term; but so too are the alternatives. Many of the problems experienced by family members before, during and after family break-up are linked to their continuing experience of conflict. If family break-up is accompanied by other changes such as a decline in material resources or a change in the physical environment, they present more problems for the family to adjust to. A requirement for optimal development is for life to be predictable and well ordered. Children and adults cope best when they know what is expected of them.

Other factors associated with the best adjustments in children in the short and medium term include: parents separated for a long time before the divorce; high socio-economic status; the child being cognitively and socially advanced and in particular having a mature understanding of conflict resolution; availability of social supports to both the parents and the children; cooperation between the parents on parenting strategies; high involvement of non-custodial parent; consistent discipline. In the longer term, being a member of a single parent family need not be problematic. The majority of children growing up in a single parent household are well adjusted and coping well, so there can be positive aspects to family break-up.

In the longer term, children often believe they have benefited from the extra responsibility they shouldered within the reduced family. They see themselves as more responsible, mature and sensitive as a result of the break-up. Family break-up can bring custodial parents and their children closer together as they come to rely increasingly on each other for emotional and social support. Children can come closer to their brothers and sisters too. This is especially likely when children are older (nine or more). One benefit of good sibling relationships at this time is they offer proof that fidelity and enduring love are possible in relationships despite the failure of their parents to achieve this. This chapter has not dealt with relationships between children and the non-custodial parent; this is addressed in the next chapter.

Family break-up can lead to growth in the separating parents, especially for women. Women who were under 30 at the time of the break-up show most gains. Amongst the benefits for women can be the impetus to develop a satisfying career which can be a source of increased self-confidence. In the long term new relationships too may prove to be more satisfying than the old one. Women frequently report that the break-up has led to an increase in confidence and in their own maturity levels (Wallerstein *et al.*, 1988).

REFERENCES

Bifulco, A.T., Brown, G.W. and Harris, T.O. (1987) Childhood loss of parents, lack of adequate parental care and adult depression: a replication, *Journal of Affective Disorders*, **12**, 115–28.
Brody, G.H. and Forehand, R. (1988) Multiple determinants of parenting: Research findings and implications for the divorce process, in E.M. Hetherington and J. Arasteh (eds.) *The Impact*

of Divorce, Single Parenting and Step-Parenting on Children, Lawrence Erlbaum Associates, New Jersey.

Camera, K.A. and Resnick, G. (1988) Interpersonal conflict and cooperation: Factors moderating children's post divorce adjustments, in E.M. Hetherington and J. Arasteh (eds.) *The Impact of Divorce, Single Parenting and Step-Parenting on Children*, Lawrence Erlbaum Associates, New Jersey.

Cummings, E.M, Iannotti, R.J. and Zahn-Waxler, C. (1985) Influence of conflict between adults on the emotions and aggression of young children, *Developmental Psychology*, **21**, 495–507.

Doherty, W.J. and Needle, R.H. (1991) Psychological adjustment and substance use among adolescents before and after a parental divorce, *Child Development*, **62**, 328–37.

Fauber, R., Forehand, R., McCombs Thomas, A. and Wierson, M. (1990) A mediational model of the impact of marital conflict on adolescent adjustment in intact and divorced families: The role of disrupted parenting, *Child Development*, **61**, 1112–23.

Furstenberg, F.F. (1988) Child care after divorce and remarriage, in E.M. Hetherington and J. Arasteh (eds.) *The Impact of Divorce, Single Parenting and Step-Parenting on Children*, Lawrence Erlbaum Associates, New Jersey.

Gorell Barnes, G. (1991) Stepfamilies in context: The post divorce process, *Association for Child Psychology and Psychiatry Newsletter*, **14**, no. 5, 3–11.

Hetherington, E.M. (1988) Parents, children and siblings: Six years after divorce, in R.A. Hinde and J. Stevenson-Hinde (eds.) *Relationships within Families: Mutual influences*, Clarendon Press, Oxford.

Hofferth, S.L. (1985) Updating children's lifecourse, *Journal of Marriage and the Family*, **47**, 93–115.

Holden, G.W. and Ritchie, K.L. (1991) Linking extreme marital discord, child rearing, and child behaviour problems: Evidence from battered women, *Child Development*, **62**, 311–27.

Kurdek, L.A. (1986) Children's reasoning about parental divorce, in R.D. Ashmore and D.M. Brodzinsky (eds.) *Thinking about the Family: Views of parents and children*, Lawrence Erlbaum Associates, New Jersey.

Wadsworth, M.E. (1985) Parenting skills and their transmission through generations, *Adoption and Fostering*, **9**, 28 –32.

Wadsworth, M.E. and Maclean, M. (1986) Parents' divorce and children's life chances, *Children and Youth Services Review*, **8**, 145–59.

Wallerstein, J.S., Corbin, S.B. and Lewis, J.M. (1988) Children of divorce: A ten year study, in E.M. Hetherington and J. Arasteh (eds.) *The Impact of Divorce, Single Parenting and Step-Parenting on Children*, Lawrence Erlbaum Associates, New Jersey.

Wicks, M. and Keirnan, K. (1990) *Family Change and Future Policy*, Joseph Rowntree Memorial Trust, London.

Zaslow, M.J. (1989) Sex differences in children's response to parental divorce: 2. Samples, variables, ages, and sources, *American Journal of Orthopsychiatry*, **59**, 118–41.

8

Reconstituted families:
step-parents and stepsiblings

David White

About 30% of children spend some part of their childhood living with a step-parent as well as one of their biological parents (White and Woollett, 1992). Families formed in this way are frequently referred to as 'reconstituted families'. This chapter will briefly examine the adjustments that have to be made when a step-parent is introduced into a family, focusing particularly on children. It will then consider some ways of helping to support children and parents in this position as well as considering some of the threats experienced by them which may require professional help.

There are many reasons why professionals may become involved with step-parent families. The incidence of depression among stepmothers is greater than for any other group of women. Child physical and sexual abuse occur more frequently among such families. Children from single parent families and step-parent families are three times as likely as children from intact homes to require professional help with psychological problems (White and Woollett, 1992). Their problem behaviours include antisocial destructive behaviours, verbal and physical aggression, poor attention span, high levels of anxiety, social withdrawal and depressed mood (Zill, 1988). They miss more time from school because of ill health and they perform less well at school academically. Furthermore, reconstituted families have a higher incidence of family break-up than other families.

A difficulty for health and welfare professionals who become involved in step-parent families and for the families themselves is that step-parent and stepchild rôles are poorly defined. Step-parents are not replacement parents, they are additional parents (Gorell Barnes, 1991). Consequently, it is unclear whether their members are expected to behave and interact together in identical ways to conventional families. Indeed, some of families' problems may stem from attempts to fit into a conventional view of a happy two-parent family rather than the more extended family form to which they actually belong.

FAMILY ADJUSTMENTS

With the introduction of a step-parent and any stepsiblings, the whole dynamics of a family change and a whole series of new relationships have to be forged and old relationships renegotiated.The formation of any new relationship calls for adjustments, but this is especially true when there are children involved and multiple adjustments have to be made by every family member. The parents have to learn to live together and develop their intimate relationships while at the same time developing and coping with their parenting rôle and the children's reactions to the new relationship. The children have to learn to share their parent's attention with the step-parent and adjust to their changing relationship with their biological parent, as they cope with their developing relationship with the step-parent. Children may also have to adjust to a changing image of their parent as a sexually active person.

In step-parent families there are competing demands set up at the same time. For the new couple the demands of parenting are hard to ignore, can take all the available time and energy and can allow too little time for the couple to be together, to be private and to get to know one another. More parents in such families report that parental relations are problematic, stressful and lack cohesion than do parents in first relationships (Bray, 1988). As a result of these extra strains, step-parent families are more prone to break-up than other families. About 10% of children experience the break-up of more than one family.

Challenges for children

Becoming part of a new family changes children's experiences; some of the changes are beneficial, some less so. The arrival of a step-parent often improves the finances of a family. With fewer worries about money parents frequently find it easier to be attentive and responsive to their children. In time a step-parent can extend the experiences of children, providing them with an additional close, stimulating and supportive relationship. They can benefit children too by the support they offer the biological parent. This support can take the form of direct help with childcare, or helping the partner indirectly by enhancing their self-esteem, making them then more calm and accessible to their children; offering advice about childcare issues; and offering reassurance that they are managing the children effectively. On these grounds a step-parent has the potential to benefit children. However the introduction of a step-parent involves changes in children's lives and changes in experience and routines can be problematic for children. They need support through the period of change.

Older children seem to be less vulnerable to change. The older children were at the initial break-up, the fewer behaviour problems they reveal when part of a step-parent family, at least until adolescence when there is an increase in reported problems. However, children aged nine to 15 years may have difficulty in adjusting to their parent's sexuality; it has been reported that they have difficulty in coping with any open sign of affection between the new couple (Hetherington, 1988).

Stepfather families

In general boys adjust to life in a stepfather family better than do girls. Within six months of remarriage boys with stepfathers show increased intellectual performance, their vocabulary increases and their arithmetic skills improve (Bray, 1988). Boys can benefit from the arrival of a stepfather, but most of the benefit comes from an improved relationship with the mother. With the formation of a new relationship the behaviour of the custodial parent to their children frequently changes. In time they usually become warmer in their interaction with their children; they also become more demanding of good and mature behaviour. Their own behaviour to their children becomes more consistent.

It takes most stepfathers quite a while to develop a sense of involvement in their stepchildren and to get used to them and to learn how best to respond to them. Initially they show little involvement, do not attempt to monitor the child's activities or to control them, make few maturity demands, interfere little and criticize little. In the first two years stepfathers report low affection for their stepchildren, but nevertheless they see themselves as working hard to present a pleasant face to their stepchildren. However stepfathers tend to be very impatient of persistent demands from their stepchildren.

Stepfathers' control of stepsons improves with the passage of time; they become more responsive and slowly become more involved in rule setting and enforcing. In turn boys become more accepting of their stepfather and they show fewer behavioural problems. In the longer term boys frequently develop a good close relationship with their stepfather and see him as supportive and seek his advice. This is most likely to occur when the mother and stepfather have developed a close relationship. In turn, the better the relationship between the parents, the more positively stepfathers feel towards their children (Brand *et al.*, 1988).

Although stepfathers can offer benefits to sons this seems to occur less frequently with daughters. Girls living with stepfathers show increased levels of distress which reveals itself both in externalizing reactions such as poor attention, aggression and overt problem behaviours, and also increased levels of internalizing reactions of anxiety, withdrawal and depression (Zaslow, 1989). The negative reactions of daughters is especially pronounced early on in the new relationship but even after two years they show unhappiness.

Within two years of the new relationship mothers have greater control over their sons but less control over their daughters. The amount of conflict with sons declines, but the conflict with daughters increases. Daughters become more demanding, hostile and coercive to both their mother and stepfather. Things improve after two years but girls are still antagonistic to both parents and are more disruptive. Not surprisingly, even after two years stepfathers find it hard to get involved with girls; they become more impatient and the number of angry exchanges between the two increases. The interactions of stepfathers and girls are very similar to those between lone mothers and sons. Stepfathers find it hard even after a long period in the family to develop good relationships with their stepdaughters. They rarely manage to establish control over them. For their part daughters see their stepfathers as unreasonable, hostile and punitive. The better the relationship between the parental couple the less secure daughters feel and the more difficult their behaviour (Bray, 1988; Brand *et al.*, 1988).

A strategy for stepfathers

The problems stepfathers encounter with their stepchildren frequently occur because stepfathers try to become involved in parenting activities too quickly with their new children. More successful stepfathers initially leave most childcare to the biological mother, only becoming involved as necessary to support the mother when her attempts at rule enforcement are failing. Gradually, as they become more accepted in the family, they begin to encourage the adoption of household rules, until after two years or so they can begin to introduce their own demands without triggering disputes.

Stepmother families

The characteristics of stepmother families differ somewhat from stepfather families and these may have a bearing on how well children adjust to this type of household. Stepmothers are more likely than stepfathers to bring their own children with them into the family, making a larger family. Additionally, stepmothers are more likely to start a family with the new partner than are mothers and stepfathers. As a result of these variations children in stepmother families are more likely to be living with stepsiblings and half-siblings. This increases the number of adjustments to be made and increases the scope for interfamily conflicts.

Unlike stepfather families, children in stepmother families show some signs of greater difficulties with long term adjustment than do children in single parent families. These children are referred more frequently for professional help for emotional, mental or behavioural problems (Zill, 1988). Children being brought up by a lone father show no more problems than children who are brought up by their mother alone, or by mothers and stepfathers. The higher incidence of behavioural problems in stepmother families is not a legacy of having spent time with a father as the single parent. The introduction of a stepmother causes children more problems than the introduction of a stepfather.

Becoming a step-parent is hard and demanding work. This is especially true for stepmothers. In most families it is the stepmother who takes over the principal child management rôle. Managing someone else's children maximizes the opportunities for disagreements and arguments. The parenting of stepmothers will be compared frequently by the children to that of the dead or departed biological mother and they will also be compared to the parenting of the father when he was the lone parent. Frequently these comparisons will be unfavourable to the stepmother, often quite unjustly, as children tend to romanticize their past experiences and to remember them as having been better than they really were. Stepmothers are seen in a more negative light by children than stepfathers, both of whom are seen as less fair and less affectionate than biological parents. Because of the demands made on stepmothers and because their efforts are not appreciated they frequently become very unhappy and can become depressed (Smith, 1990). It would seem that the introduction of a stepfather presents different adjustment challenges to children than the introduction of a stepmother.

Several studies show that while boys are equally happy with stepmothers and stepfathers during the early years of the new family, it is again girls who have particular difficulties, revealing more aggressive behaviours or becoming more inhibited (e.g. Brand *et al.*, 1988). If the stepmother can establish good relations with her stepdaughter then the girl makes better adjustments. It is suggested that one reason why girls can experience particular difficulties with the introduction of a step-parent is that they lose some of their prestige within the family. When the family is a single parent family girls frequently are asked to take on extra responsibility for household tasks and for looking after younger siblings. Moreover, they frequently form close relationships with the lone parent. With the introduction of a step-parent their special rôle within the family is undermined and they have to share their parent's attention with the step-parent. This frequently results in resentment and hostility directed not only at the step-parent but also towards the biological parent.

A strategy for stepmothers

Gorell Barnes (1991) has pointed out that for fathers to have custody of children, it is likely that the relationship between those children and their biological mother was unsatisfactory. Subsequently when they become a part of a stepmother family the earlier problematic relationship may interfere with the new relationship with the stepmother. It may be easier for stepmothers to cope with hostility from stepchildren if they can recognize that they may not be the direct cause of that behaviour but the recipient of the stepchildren's unresolved difficulties with their biological mother. Stepmothers can rarely adopt the strategy open to stepfathers of maintaining an initial distance between themselves and their stepchildren. Consequently they need to be much more flexible in their approach, trying different approaches, monitoring their own and their children's behaviour and selecting strategies that work best for them. In the long term stepmothers' relationships with their stepchildren generally improve.

SUPPORTS AND THREATS TO CHILDREN WITHIN STEP-PARENT FAMILIES

Life for children can be enhanced by their experiences in a step-parent family but sometimes their experiences can threaten their well-being. In this final section the darker as well as the brighter side of life in a step-parent family will be considered.

Break-up of step-parent families

If the new reconstituted family remains together, each member can benefit in the long term from the support offered to them by the new family members and by changes for the better in their relations with the existing family. However if the family does not remain together the repeated experience of family break-up can be damaging. Unfortunately, the demands made on a couple by children can allow them insufficient time and energy to solve any initial interpersonal problems in their relationship. Moreover hostility from children may be so unpleasant as to swamp any pleasures that the adults might otherwise have found in each other's company. Because step-parent families on average are less cohesive than average first-time families, conflict occurs frequently. Causes for conflict include the behaviour of the children, how to respond to the children and money spent on children.

Conflict between the couple can swing the balance against continuing the relationship and step-parent families break up more frequently than other families. This can add considerably to the stress experienced by family members. Children have to make repeated adjustments, first to the initial break-up, then to the new relationship, then to the second break-up. The deleterious effect of the first break-up is added to the negative effects of the remarriage of a parent. Marital or relationship transitions show cumulative effects (Furstenberg and Seltzer, 1986). Consequently children who undergo repeated family changes begin to show more marked effects. Each marital transition takes its toll on children, leading to slight increases in children's sense of insecurity and slight deterioration in their sense of well-being.

Child abuse

Step-parent families, just like other families, may have periods when conflicts between members occur. Sometimes this escalates into more serious forms when a parent or step-parent physically abuses their children. While the majority of step-parent families are *not* involved in child abuse, physical abuse is somewhat more common in step-parent and especially stepfather families than in other families. A second form of child abuse that occurs more commonly in step-parent families is child sexual abuse. Frequently both these forms of abuse go together: for example, a child may be beaten to ensure their silence about sexual abuse. In some families, abuse affects only one child whereas in others all the children are abused.

Physical abuse

Both men and women physically abuse children; mothers, step-mothers, fathers and stepfathers could all be involved if this form of abuse occurs in step-parent families. Physical abuse is most likely to occur during periods when the relationship be-tween parents is at a low ebb. Because step-parent families are often less cohesive than other families there can be more argu-ments resulting in an increased incidence of physical abuse. Stepfathers often have little experience of children and so they may have unrealistic expectations of young children's behavi-our and misperceive their stepchild as being out of control and in need of firm discipline. When this type of belief is coupled with characteristics such as low self-esteem, depression, hostility and low tolerance of frustration, it can result in insensitive parent-ing, an inability to put the child's needs before their own and at worst inappropriate and punitive behaviour (Browne *et al.*, 1988).

Boys, younger children and handicapped children are more likely to be abused than others. Boys are more at risk, in part, because when they are unhappy they are more likely to show their distress by exhibiting highly visible negative behaviours such as whining, refusing requests and increased aggression. In contrast girls are more likely to conceal their distress, to become more withdrawn, anxious and depressed (Zaslow, 1989). For a parent who is feeling stressed the negative behaviour of boys is much more irritating than the withdrawn behaviour of girls and is much more likely to elicit hostility. Continued negativity in boys may aggravate or escalate parents' anger and aggres-sion. This is particularly marked for step-parents whose inter-actions with stepchildren are frequently described as corrosive (Browne *et al.*, 1988). Similarly younger children are more likely than older children to whine or have temper tantrums in trying to get their own way and so irritate parents. Handicapped children make different demands on parents but again are highly demanding of them. When parents are stressed this may irritate them and elicit more hostile responses.

Helping parents who abuse

Assistance can be given to parents and step-parents who abuse their children physically. Since parents and step-parents who have a good relationship together feel more positively about their children and consequently respond to them more sensitively and less punitively, this offers one route for interventions: through counselling to provide information about conflict resolution, intimacy and sexual issues. A second, complementary approach is to concentrate more on helping abusing parents and step-parents develop more realistic understandings of their children, their capabilities and the appropriateness of their behaviour. Often abusing parents are isolated from other parents and so have no opportunity to share experiences and to see their own children's behaviour in context. By providing them with the opportunity to talk about what irritates and upsets them, professionals can help the parents to an understanding of what is appropriate and acceptable behaviour in children and how they can best deal with naughtiness and their own angry reactions to it.

Sexual abuse

The majority of cases of sexual abuse involves girls and children of all ages may be victims (see Chapter 9). Most sexual abusers are male, so when sexual abuse occurs within step-parent families stepfathers and sometimes stepbrothers are involved. Family life throws children, stepfathers and stepbrothers into close and intimate proximity. This can offer frequent opportunities for sexual abuse to occur (La Fontaine, 1990). It can also provide privacy, even from other family members, especially when those family members do not want to face up to the possibility. A mother who has struggled to rear her children as a single parent, who has felt lonely and isolated during that period, but who has now found intimacy and support from a new partner has a strong incentive for overlooking what evidence there may be.

Even when abuse is suspected, disclosure can be costly for the whole family including the victim of abuse. Reporting the abuse can lead to the prosecution and imprisonment of the abuser and to the disintegration of the family. A series of relationships that are working well may be terminated and members of the family may see their chances of happiness receding. Mothers and siblings may be angry with the victims in these circumstances and blame them for what has happened and perhaps believe that they have encouraged the sexual activities that have taken place. Concern for their own happiness and beliefs about the victim's contribution to the situation can provide mothers and others with an incentive for helping to conceal what has been happening.

Tackling sexual abuse

There is considerable debate about the best ways to deal with abuse. Prosecuting abusers and putting children into care may stop the abuse and punish abusers but may in themselves create yet more problems for children and the rest of the family. A better solution may be to seek ways of supporting families and trying to improve parent-child relations (Browne *et al.*, 1988).

When stepfathers or stepbrothers sexually abuse children they are ignoring children's feelings or they are assuming that the children view the activities in the same way that they do. This misperception can be reinforced if children appear to enjoy their special relationship with stepfathers or stepbrothers and the extra attention they get (Browne *et al.*, 1988). It has been suggested that one way of preventing abuse is for stepfathers to get more involved in childcare, so they get to know their children as individuals in their own right and so become more sensitive to their children's needs and to their signals and can come to recognize that their beliefs about the child are distorted. By establishing close relationships, stepfathers may respect children more and be less likely to use them for their own sexual purposes and become more sensitive to children's expressions of fear, reluctance or dislike of what they are asked to do (White and Woollett, 1992).

Contact with the absent biological parent

Children in step-parent families may have contact still with their absent biological parent. Following the introduction of a step-parent into the family the absent parent tends to reduce their contact with the children. This is especially true of visits to girls. Both non-custodial mothers and fathers are more likely to maintain contact with sons (Brand *et al.*, 1988), and non-custodial mothers are better at maintaining contact than non-custodial fathers. The longer the duration of the step-parent family the less frequent the visits from the non-custodial parent. However, some non-custodial parents continue to visit and show an interest in their children. This may or may not be a source of support for children. If they do see their biological parent regularly this could influence their relationship with both the custodial parent and the step-parent. If a child is seeing their absent biological parent this can introduce loyalty conflicts. By enjoying the contact with the biological parent they may seem to be betraying the step-parent. If there is still hostility between the two biological parents then contact with the absent biological parent may also be associated with increased conflict.

In general it appears that children cope quite happily with two father figures in their lives. Children's overt behaviours are not affected by continued contact with their biological father; they are no worse and no better. However, having two mother figures appears to be more problematic. In stepmother families regular contact with the biological mother is associated with poor child-stepmother relations. Girls especially find it easier to form good relations with their stepmother if they are not in regular contact with their biological mother; in these cases there is less conflict of loyalties (Brand *et al.*, 1988). If their biological mother has died children find it easier to accept a substitute than when the biological mother still lives, and this is true whether or not they have contact with their biological mother. Least satisfaction with a stepmother occurs when a child is in regular contact with their biological mother. The acceptance of stepfathers is not influenced by these considerations, reflecting their more peripheral rôle in most households. Clearly dynamics do vary from family to family, but continued contact with the non-custodial parent can pose problems for the developing relationship with the step-parent and in particular with a stepmother.

Although continuing contact with the departed parent can cause problems within the step-parent family, children usually prefer to maintain contact. Clinical evidence suggests that it is important not to shut out any mention of the departed parent. It is important for children that the memories of their biological parents are maintained and that they are allowed to construct a meaningful picture of their family and of family relationships. Equally it is important for the successful absorption of step-parents into families that they develop a rôle that is complementary to that of the absent parent, rather than denying the existence of that parent (Gorell Barnes, 1991).

Other relationships in the family

The introduction of a step-parent into the family changes relationships within the immediate and extended family. The way in which siblings get on may be affected. Early in the life of the new family girls are especially distant from their siblings. So not only do they turn away from their biological parent, and reject their step-parent, but they also avoid their siblings; they cut themselves off from the whole family. It is not only girls who have difficulty interacting with their siblings following the arrival of a step-parent; relationships involving boys also tend to be problematic early on, but girls show this to a more marked degree. If sibling relations are to improve it is important that parents are fair and consistent in their treatment of all children, otherwise rivalries develop. If parents treat one child with less warmth and affection and greater restrictiveness than another, that sibling is likely to be more aggressive and unaffectionate to their siblings. Consistent good parental treatment is associated with good sibling relationships.

Consistency is even more important when there are stepsiblings and half-siblings. Their presence clearly increases the number of new relationships to be formed and provides enormous scope for personality clashes, conflicts, perceived injustices and other sources of renewed family tension. In many households this would appear to happen and the presence of a stepsibling or half-sibling is associated with more behavioural problems in children. Children are happiest when they do not have to share their biological parent's attention with other new children.

Becoming part of a step-parent family can change contact with the extended family. Following the introduction of a step-parent children typically see less of their grandparents. Frequently lone parents live with their own parents and the formation of a new relationship can mean a reduction in contact with the custodial grandparents. Additionally, the grandparents on the non-custodial parent's side frequently cease contact. However, although contact with biological grandparents may decline a new extended family is frequently introduced in the form of the parents and relations of the

step-parent. Stepgrandparents are frequently enthusiastic
about their new rôle. For their part, children up to the age of
adolescence tend to be very accepting of these new
steprelatives. Changing relationships within the family can
provide support and help children make their adjustments, but
they can also add to the stress of adjusting to a step-parent
family. For all family members, having access to supportive
family and friendship networks is of great value.

CONCLUSION

The introduction of a step-parent calls for adjustments from all
family members that can be problematic in the short term. For
most children the middle term effects are minor; academically
they do slightly worse, they are slightly more troublesome to
their parents and at school. There can be definite longer term
advantages to children in these families if they last. The
educational attainment of children in step-parent families
is better than that of children from single parent families and
the improved socio-economic status of the reconstituted
family improves children's socio-economic status as adults.
Step-parent families can become cohesive, providing supportive environments offering security and close relationships
for all the family, but achieving this environment requires time
and patience.

Unfortunately this cohesive environment is not always
achieved and family members may develop problems requiring
professional assistance. Step-parents who fail to recognize or
respond to the needs of their stepchildren place increased
stresses upon them, which in turn can lead to increasingly
corrosive relationships in the family that in extreme cases result
in abusive as well as insensitive behaviour. When a reconstituted family follows on from family break-up, step-parents may
fail to recognize the problems that family members have as a
result of the earlier break-up and so be insufficiently sympathetic to the needs and demands of their new family. Furthermore they may erroneously attribute difficulties in family
relationships to a personal antagonism to their own presence
and so feel rejected and undervalued. Recognition of these
possible dynamics is useful for those who become involved in
supporting members of step-parent families.

REFERENCES

Brand, E., Clingempeel, W.G. and Bowen-Woodward, K. (1988) Family relationships and children's psychological adjustment in stepmother and stepfather families, in E.M. Hetherington and J. Arasteh (eds.) *The Impact of Divorce, Single Parenting and Step-Parenting on Children*, Lawrence Erlbaum Associates, New Jersey.

Bray, J.H. (1988) Children's development during early remarriage, in E.M. Hetherington and J. Arasteh (eds.) *The Impact of Divorce, Single Parenting and Step-Parenting on Children*, Lawrence Erlbaum Associates, New Jersey.

Browne, K., Davies, C. and Stratton, P. (1988) *Early Prediction and Prevention of Child Abuse*, Wiley, Chichester.

Furstenberg, F.F. and Seltzer, J.A. (1986) Divorce and child development, in P.A. Adler and P. Adler (eds.) *Sociological Studies of Child Development, Vol. 1*, JAI Press, London.

Gorell Barnes, G. (1991) Stepfamilies in context: The post divorce process, *Association for Child Psychology and Psychiatry Newsletter*, **14**, no. 5, 3–11.

Hetherington, E.M. (1988) Parents, children and siblings six years after divorce, in R. Hinde and J. Stevenson-Hinde (eds.) *Relationships within Families: Mutual influences*, Clarendon Press, Oxford.

La Fontaine, J. (1990) *Child Sexual Abuse*, Polity Press, Cambridge.

Smith, D. (1990) *Stepmothering*, Harvester Wheatsheaf, Hemel Hempstead.

White, D. and Woollett, A. (1992) *Families: A context for development*, Falmer Press, Basingstoke.

Zaslow, M.J. (1989) Sex differences in children's response to parental divorce: 2. Samples, variables, ages, and sources, *American Journal of Orthopsychiatry*, **59**, 118–41.

Zill, N. (1988) Behaviour, achievement, and health problems among children in stepfamilies: Findings from a national survey of child health, in E.M. Hetherington and J. Arasteh (eds.) *The Impact of Divorce, Single Parenting and Step-Parenting on Children*, Lawrence Erlbaum Associates, New Jersey.

9

Child sexual abuse

Stephen Frosh

INTRODUCTION: REAL EVENTS AND MORAL PANICS

For several years, child sexual abuse has been a major focus of concern for professionals dealing with children. Its power to panic, confuse and immobilize is profound, as is its capacity to attract attention and generate emotive debate. Some people have been able to enhance their careers by means of their expertise in investigating or working with sexually abused children; other careers have been broken by mistakes or by 'moral panics' – outbursts of anger or displaced blame against professionals, often containing an unmistakably hysterical quality (Levidow, 1989).

All professionals working in this area are repeatedly faced with dilemmas and anguishing, unresolvable uncertainties. Has a child been abused or not? Why will a child not speak about her or his abusive experiences when everyone 'knows' they have occurred? Why are so many 'disclosures' later retracted? Why do professionals so often differ heatedly amongst themselves when discussing whether sexual abuse has occurred, how to find out if it has, and what kind of action to take? Why are relatively inexperienced staff so often left unsupported, facing the most awkward and sensitive of situations, apparently alone? And why, when people often seem so certain about what is right in theory, does it seem to be impossible to know what to do when faced with an actual case?

Clearly, the sexual abuse of children strikes hard at some core assumptions and emotions, challenging social beliefs and also exposing a troubling underside to our apparent concern for the welfare of children. Physical abuse can, of course, be just as troubling and emotive: witness the attacks on social work competence that have accompanied several famous cases

(Parton, 1985). However, the additional factor of sex makes child sexual abuse perhaps uniquely disturbing, or at least disturbing in a unique way. The reluctance of professionals and lay people alike to recognize the existence of sexual abuse is well documented (e.g. Campbell, 1989), as is the eagerness with which its existence is denied. The characteristic secrecy and uncertainty of sexual abuse (only about 50% of sexually abused children have associated physical signs, and these are generally regarded as 'compatible with', rather than specific to, such abuse: Glaser, 1992) make the denial of its reality that much easier, for abusers and observers alike.

Secrecy and sexuality: these dual features constantly plague professionals working with sexually abused children. Often, it is not possible to establish with certainty that a child has been sexually abused; one has to continue to live in doubt, making probability judgements, setting up channels through which a child could communicate about her or his abuse if she or he so wishes, tolerating the possibility that a child might have to be left in an abusing situation until she or he is ready to speak out. Always, there is the disturbance of sex, of dealing with one's own sexuality, of recognizing and managing what might be precociously sexualized behaviour on the part of the child (who may have a wider range of sexual experiences than the adult worker), and of dealing with other people's voyeuristic fantasies. In this quagmire, keeping one's professional balance is an exceedingly difficult task.

This chapter can offer only a brief overview of some of the major issues involved in work with sexually abused children. In keeping with a generally 'psychological' framework, the focus will not be on procedural, statutory or legal issues, but on the behavioural, emotional and relational considerations which need to be taken into account. First, however, some background factors need to be outlined – particularly issues of definition, the frequency and common characteristics of sexual abuse, and its probable effects.

DEFINING CHILD SEXUAL ABUSE

A number of alternative definitions of child sexual abuse have been employed in the literature, the best known being that offered by Schechter and Roberge (1976):

'...the involvement of dependent, developmentally immature children and adolescents in sexual activities they do not
truly comprehend, to which they are unable to give informed
consent, or that violate the social taboos of family roles.'

(p. 60)

This definition serves well for most practical purposes, even
though it does not specify any of its terms – for example, what
is meant by 'developmentally immature' or 'sexual'. Its principal strengths are that it recognizes that children are in dependent positions with respect to adults and that it separates the
concept of abuse from that of harm; that is, it is not necessary
to establish that a child has been harmed in order for a certain
act to be designated as abusive. What is required is, centrally,
that the child should be 'unable to give informed consent', a
criterion which is perhaps tautological with that of the child
being 'developmentally immature'.

An important caveat to definitions such as that given above,
in which an attempt is made to include all sexually abusive acts,
is offered by Haugaard and Reppucci (1988). They argue that,
particularly for research purposes, finer distinctions between
different types and contexts of abuse are necessary. For
example, they write:

'Phrases that are relatively specific, such as *children molested
by their parents*, or even more specific, such as *adolescents who
have had intercourse with their fathers*, provide much more
meaningful information than does *child sexual abuse victims*.'

(p. 30)

Overall, however, for practical purposes, the central issues – the
central components of child sexual abuse – are the involvement
of children (usually legally defined as aged 16 years or less) by
people in a position of power over them (including all adults)
in sexual activities.

THE FREQUENCY OF CHILD SEXUAL ABUSE

Investigations of the frequency with which children are
sexually abused have produced a fairly wide range of figures, largely as a consequence of the use of differing sample
populations and differing definitions of abuse. The number of

suspected and established cases of sexual abuse referred to statutory and treatment agencies has increased enormously in the last decade, at a rate in the USA of over 10% per year (Finkelhor, 1991) and with a possibly even higher rate of increase in the UK. These, however, are already selected cases in that they have overcome some very powerful hurdles to recognition: for example, suspicion, partial disclosure, informing authorities, responses on the part of the authorities. Population surveys, in which relatively large samples of the general population are asked whether they have been sexually abused in the past, provide more comprehensive information about the frequency of abuse – although it should be noted that this refers to *past* rather than current rates of abuse. That is, as these surveys usually work by asking adults about their experiences of being sexually abused, they provide information on the proportion of adults who were sexually abused in childhood, but not the current 'incidence' rates.

The best available estimate of child sexual abuse in the UK population comes from Baker and Duncan (1985), whose investigation involved an interview of 2019 British women and men aged 15+ years in a nationally representative sample. They provided interviewees with a broad definition of sexual abuse ('A child [anyone under 16 years] is sexually abused when another person, who is sexually mature, involves the child in any activity which the other person expects to lead to their sexual arousal') and asked if this had happened to them in childhood. Twelve percent of female and 8% of male interviewees responded affirmatively, whilst a further 13% of the sample refused to answer. Of the abused sample, 49% had experienced 'contact' abuse (i.e. some form of physical contact was involved), 51% 'non-contact' (exhibitionism, voyeurism, etc.). These figures seem very high, but they are similar to those of some comparable international studies (e.g. Mullen *et al.*, 1988, in New Zealand) and are actually lower than those found in the USA (e.g. Russell, 1983).

Baker and Duncan's (1985) finding that women were one-and-a-half times as likely as men to report having been sexually abused in childhood is in line with the general findings of other surveys, which suggest that girls are abused approximately twice as often as boys. These findings, however, contradict those obtained from studies of *identified* sexually abused children, in which girls predominate over boys at a rate of four or five to one (Finkelhor, 1991; Haugaard and Reppucci, 1988). This discrepancy suggests that the blocks to disclosure of sexual abuse when the victim is male may be even greater than when the victim is female. One consequence of this is that many abused boys only come to the attention of professionals when they themselves abuse others (Bentovim, 1991); more generally, the need to address openly a child's possible anxieties about disclosure are even more compelling with boys than with girls.

The gender distribution of *abusers* is also the subject of some dispute, with earlier studies suggesting that 90 to 99% of abusers of girls and 40 to 97% of boys are male (Haugaard and Reppucci, 1988). More recent studies suggest that these figures may underestimate the frequency of abuse by women; it is, nevertheless, still clear that the large majority of abusers are male. The implications of this fact for preventive and treatment programmes have been widely discussed (e.g. Glaser and Frosh, 1988; Frosh, 1988; MacLeod and Sarraga, 1988). True primary prevention requires programmes focusing on the development of masculine sexuality and its characteristic separation from the expression of intimate and dependent feelings; in treatment contexts, the likely gender associations of abuse in the mind of victims need to be taken into consideration, in particular when making decisions about whether to use male or female therapists.

Also on the subject of abusers, it appears that the majority of sexual abusers are previously known to their child victims, although there is more stranger-abuse of boys than of girls (Russell, 1983; Baker and Duncan, 1985). However, the stereotypical notion that most abuse is incestuous abuse by fathers or stepfathers is also not accurate – much is by other relatives, family friends or other adults in positions of power over the children concerned (Haugaard and Reppucci, 1988). It also appears that single occurrences of abuse are most common, but a substantial minority are abused over a period of time (e.g. 63% of the abused sample in Baker and Duncan's 1985 study reported only being abused once, 23% reported repeated abuse by the same person and 14% reported multiple abuse). Only a minority of abusive encounters involve full sexual intercourse (about 5%), although oral and anal intercourse are common, especially when the victims are boys or young girls. The most common reported sexual activity in surveys is genital or non-genital fondling.

THE EFFECTS OF CHILD SEXUAL ABUSE

There is now considerable evidence that child sexual abuse is generally harmful to the children concerned, although there is substantial variation in the extent of this harm. Reports from clinical samples show that, in childhood, sexual abuse is associated with depression, feelings of guilt, lowered self-esteem, phobias, nightmares, bedwetting, sexualized behaviour, school refusal, adolescent pregnancies and suicide attempts – the whole gamut of mild, moderate and severe childhood disturbances. In the longer term, having been abused as a child is linked in adulthood particularly to impaired self-esteem, especially sexual self-esteem, depression, suicide attempts, anxiety and drug and alcohol addiction (Haugaard and Reppucci, 1988; Glaser and Frosh, 1988; Berliner, 1991). Reports from general population samples also reveal characteristically negative effects of child sexual abuse, but, as one might expect, with more variability in their magnitude. Haugaard and Reppucci (1988, p. 75) note:

'Whereas the clinical samples consisted almost exclusively of those suffering relatively serious negative consequences, the empirical evidence included some abuse victims who suffered no apparent consequences.'

Berliner (1991) surveys evidence to suggest that:

'While abused children as a group are consistently found to have more problems than children who have not been abused, in general they do not have as many problems as children who are identified in psychiatric populations. In all of the recent studies, not even 50 per cent of the children achieved clinically significant levels of distress on the direct assessment measures.'

(p. 147)

In the longer term, too:

'Approximately 80 per cent of cases in the research studies do not result in psychiatric diagnosis in adult survivors.'

(p. 148)

Nevertheless, Berliner again lists several studies that have revealed very significantly raised levels of distress and risk for psychiatric disorder in adult survivors, making it clear that despite this variation in outcome, the risks to mental health caused by sexual abuse in childhood are very substantial.

Numerous factors probably act together to determine the severity of the effects of sexual abuse. Those best established in the research literature are the following:

1. Prior emotional health: positive previous psychological well-being is a protective factor;
2. Duration of abuse: the longer the duration, the worse the consequences seem to be;
3. Relationship with abuser: the closer the relationship, the worse the outcome appears to be;
4. Type of abuse: the more intrusive the sexual contact (e.g. intercourse versus exhibitionism), the worse the outcome;
5. Response to abuse: the more supportive the response on the part of surrounding adults, the better the outcome.

This last factor may be the most important; a 'supportive response' is often selected by adult survivors as the main thing they were looking for (and frequently failed to receive) when disclosing their abuse for the first time (Moore, 1991). While the receptiveness of professionals to children's allegations of abuse has improved enormously in recent years, it is still the case that the complications of disclosure work, particularly when possible criminal prosecution is at issue, may interfere with the provision of a genuinely supportive response and – possibly even more to the point – may lead children to expect an interrogation rather than a hearing should they indeed disclose. The development of supportive and yet evidentially acceptable contexts for disclosure is a major professional task; in practice, this very often means that professionals who suspect that a child is being abused need to consider very carefully who might be the most helpful person to talk with that child, and in what setting.

Finkelhor (1988) has proposed a model of 'Four Traumatogenic Dynamics' to account for the impact of sexual abuse on a child's psychological state, these being: (a) traumatic sexualization; (b) betrayal of trust; (c) stigmatization or blame; (d) powerlessness. This model has received quite widespread acceptance amongst researchers and clinicians alike, although

Glaser (1992) argues that it requires the addition of two further dynamics for completeness. These are, first, the sense of fear and isolation produced by the secrecy that characterizes sexual abuse, and secondly, the confusion which most or all sexually abused children experience: 'They are confronted by sexual activities whose meaning and purpose they cannot fully, if at all, comprehend; unpleasant sensations are silently evoked by the actions of loving adults; "naughty" and "rude" behaviour is perpetrated by trusted persons' (p. 8).

In summary, although there is considerable variation in the response to sexual abuse shown by different children, there is no doubt that abuse acts as a significant stressor and substantially raises the risk of childhood or later adult psychological difficulties. The sources of this raised risk probably lie in a mixture of the specific sexual content of the abuse and the general context of betrayal of trust, secrecy and powerlessness. Perhaps above all else, sexually abused children seek non-blaming, supportive responses from adults. Indeed, it may be their prediction of the likelihood that this is what they will find that decides whether or not they willingly disclose what has happened to them.

INDICATORS OF CHILD SEXUAL ABUSE

All the major professions involved in work with children now have set procedures for dealing with suspicions or claims of sexual abuse. Even the best of these procedures, however, cannot remove the uncertainty that is endemic to identification of abuse, and indeed a good deal of the time of many professionals is taken up with assessing claims or suspicions that particular children have been abused. There are many indirect indicators of sexual abuse, for example sexualized behaviour, unusual avoidance of men, hints of secrets, or physical signs compatible with sexual abuse. By its nature, however, such evidence is inconclusive, because it may have other explanations. With the exception of a small number of children on whom there is incontrovertible physical evidence, it is only when a child and/or an abuser reveals that abuse has occurred that one can be completely sure. In this respect, it is worth noting that the most recent evidence supports the contention that it is unusual for children to make false allegations of sexual abuse, even in the context of divorce and custody proceedings (Myers *et al.*,

1989). Abusers, on the other hand, commonly deny that abuse has occurred, or deny the abusive meaning of any established sexual contact (Glaser and Frosh, 1988). Therefore, if a child makes a clear disclosure, it is a reasonable rule of thumb that abuse is likely to have taken place, whatever the alleged abuser might say. On the other hand, it is frequently the case that the child's 'disclosure' is by no means clear, or is retracted at a later date, leaving all the professionals in an extremely uncomfortable state of not knowing, perhaps for evermore.

Overall, it is important to recognize that children are often in a 'double-bind' when faced with the dilemma of whether or not to disclose what is happening – fear of the consequences if they do not (e.g. continued abuse, abuse of a sibling by the same abuser), fear of the consequences if they do (e.g. family break-up, prison for a loved father, being taken into care, being blamed). It should surprise no-one, therefore, that uncertainty is endemic to this area; too quick and definite assertions about what *must* have happened should always be avoided. What are often the most important professional tasks are, first, the maintenance of good links between everyone involved with a child and, second, the setting up of structures for observation and response that will make it possible to act supportively and coherently if the child does at some point speak of being abused or, at least, if more indirect evidence of abuse becomes available. The ability to live in doubt in this very emotive and painful area of work is a significant professional skill.

THE THERAPEUTIC NEEDS OF SEXUALLY ABUSED CHILDREN

This section is based on the outline in Glaser and Frosh (1988) of the 'post-validation' (i.e. after the establishment of the fact of sexual abuse) needs of sexually abused children. In that outline, we articulate the aim of a therapeutically oriented (rather than purely investigative) intervention as follows:

> 'Comforting and making sense of bewilderment, confusion and anger. It is also concerned with protection for the child and with changes that may offer new experiences in relationships and an improvement in self-image for individuals.'

> (p.110)

The focus is thus on the interests of the child rather than on those of others (e.g. the family or the abuser); however, there is often strong justification for intervention in the wider context in order to meet the child's needs.

The following considerations should be taken into account when assessing the post-validation therapeutic needs of sexually abused children.

Protection of the child's sexuality

Within the family

The simple act of disclosure is insufficient to prevent re-abuse, as it is clear that, particularly in intrafamilial situations in which abuse is part of a network of pre-existing relationships, re-abuse by the same person is a not uncommon phenomenon. Probably the only reliable way to prevent this is to ensure continued separation of the child and the abuser; always, it is necessary to assess the ability of the non-abusing parent(s) to protect the child. Factors that might inhibit such protectiveness include the continuing need of the non-abusing parent for a relationship with the abuser (e.g. if the abuser is the husband or father of the parent) and possibly internal factors such as anger or guilt directed at the child. In this respect, however, it is worth noting that, contrary to many stereotypes and indeed to the expectations of many abused children, the vast majority of mothers (70%) believe their child when disclosure occurs (Jones, 1991).

Protection from new sexual abuse

The same issues of protection arise here as above, with the added factor that the premature sexualization of children implicit in sexual abuse may make abused children more vulnerable to other potential abusers. This is particularly the case when a child has experienced the sexual abuse as possessing some positive characteristics, for instance as feeling pleasant physically, or as the only context in which intimate care was expressed for them. The various preventive programmes teaching 'good sense defence' and other resistance and assertiveness skills (e.g. Kidscape, 1986) have a contribution to make here, although they have not been very extensively evaluated and run the risk of encouraging children to mistakenly believe that they are responsible for protecting themselves from abuse, and powerful enough actually so to do.

Protection from inappropriate sexual involvement with other children

Some abused children re-enact or mimic the abuse they have experienced, leading to rejection and humiliation by other children and also, at times, to abuse of younger children (cf. the evidence that a significant number of adolescent sexual offenders have themselves been sexually abused (Pierce and Pierce, 1987)). Working with these children on appropriate boundaries of trust and consent – central areas of transgression in sexually abusive acts – and on related issues such as ownership of one's body and sex education is an important form of intervention, perhaps most usefully carried out in group settings (Hildebrand, 1989).

The child's emotions

As noted earlier, confusion and a sense of guilt mixed with anger seem to be common consequences of the abusive experience for a child (as indeed they often are for other family members and professionals themselves). The extent to which the child's emotions are in turmoil varies greatly from child to child, presumably as a function of the vulnerability factors described above. In addition, the sexual feelings provoked by the abuse may be difficult to deal with, as may be a child's continuing ambivalent feelings towards the abuser (love as well as hate) or anger at a perceived lack of protection from the parent (e.g. Herman (1981) found that girls who had been abused by their fathers sometimes felt more immediate anger towards their mothers for not protecting them than towards the abusers themselves). In this context, the enormous uncertainties of police and court procedures can add substantially to a child's emotional distress.

The family context

Family assessment and treatment in child sexual abuse has

often been thought of as centring on the attribution of responsibility for the abuse and the potential rehabilitation of abusers
into the family. Although this does indeed form part of child
sexual abuse work (e.g. Bentovim *et al.*, 1989), it is more common for professionals to be dealing with families in which the
abuser is not resident, either because he has left or because he
was never a member of the immediate family anyway. In those
circumstances, there are various issues concerning the impact
of the abuse and its discovery on the family which may become
central to the post-validation professional task.

Protective capacity of the family

This has been dealt with above: to what extent can this family
be relied upon, or worked with, in order to ensure the protection of the child from further abuse?

Mother (non-abusing parent) – child relationship

There is a large array of possible stressors to deal with here,
from relationship difficulties predating the abuse or its disclosure, to the child's anger at the mother for not offering protection. If a mother has been sexually abused in childhood herself
(as will be the case in something up to 20% of instances even if
sexual abuse in the mothers of abused children is no more
common than in the general population), there may be special
difficulties for her in dealing with what has happened to her
child. The aim of intervention is to facilitate clear communication of feelings while also (a) protecting the child against parental anger or against having to carry the burden of a mother's
distress, and (b) encouraging the mother to accept the child's
emotions. This may well require preliminary individual work
with the mother.

Abuser – child relationship

This is an area of great difficulty. There are no cast-iron guarantees against re-abuse, even if an abuser accepts responsibility
for what has happened and even if he serves a prison sentence.
From the point of view of the child, it is most important to allow

142 *Child sexual abuse*

the expression and management of ambivalent feelings in the context of a clear statement of the abuser's responsibility for what has happened. If an abuser who has been in a longstanding relationship with the child (e.g. a father or stepfather) can explicitly acknowledge the abusive nature of the sexual contact, this may offer the child confirmation of her or his worth and entitlement to feelings of anger and betrayal.

Non-abusing parent – abuser relationship

It may be that this is the most important assessment area when considering the viability of a child's continued placement in her or his family. A non-abusing parent who cannot extricate her or himself from a relationship with an abuser is less likely to be able to offer protection to the child and more likely to doubt the child's word or role in the abuse, even if the initial response to disclosure had been belief and support. Complicated situations such as when a mother has been abused in the past by her own father who then abuses her child (his grandchild) may be particularly difficult to resolve.

Siblings

The possibility that siblings of an abused child may themselves have been abused will always need to be considered. In addition, siblings may have been fully or partially aware of the existence of continuing abuse but may not have disclosed it themselves, leaving them with their own feelings of guilt or confusion to deal with. They may also harbour resentment towards the abused child or the child protection services for apparently being responsible for breaking up the family home – especially if the siblings are natural children of a father who has been abusing his stepchild.

Substitute families and children in residential care

When abused children do have to be taken into care, this is sometimes experienced as a relief but it may also be felt as proof of their own guilt or badness. They may require special counselling to deal with these feelings. The substitute families themselves will almost certainly require support in dealing with sexually abused children, for example around issues such as managing sexualized behaviour or explaining to other children in the family what the particular history of the abused child has been. Staff in residential children's homes are often faced with very difficult, acting-out children and are possibly in a very vulnerable position; both children and staff in such settings routinely require professional back-up.

THERAPEUTIC INTERVENTIONS

The previous section identified a number of different concerns which might face a professional wishing to offer a therapeutic response to a sexually abused child and her or his family. There is a range of ways in which attempts to deal with these have been made, although it is fair to note that there is rather little by way of convincing empirical evidence for the effectiveness of any of them. In summary, however, the main options available are the following.

Group therapy

Group therapy possesses the advantage of providing a setting in which experiences can be shared in a contained and relatively safe way, thus counteracting the secrecy and sense of isolation which is otherwise characteristic of sexual abuse. It may also offer peer support and a wide variety of emotional and coping strategies for group members. On the other hand, groups can be very difficult to set up, as they usually require a reasonable level of homogeneity of age and experience amongst the members; the consequence can be that children or carers referred for group therapy have to wait an inordinately long time before the group actually takes place. Even with this precaution, some members of a group may find it less relevant or useful than others; collusive avoidance of important issues and maladaptive learning can also sometimes occur.

With these caveats, however, there is considerable clinical experience with groups of abused children and with groups of carers suggesting the value of this kind of work, both in its own right and as an assessment procedure for further intensive psychotherapy in some cases (Hildebrand, 1989).

Family therapy

Family therapy, usually without but occasionally with the abuser, has a significant assessment function in both child protection and emotional needs contexts. Therapeutically, it is a particularly powerful way of addressing issues of secrecy and communication, scapegoating, blame and responsibility. It can offer a space for work with siblings and deal with inter-generational issues in a live and concrete way. Perhaps most importantly, engaging in family therapy embodies the statement that the sexual abuse of one member and its disclosure has consequences for the family as a whole system: consequences such as dealing with anger and guilt, with the practical impact of child protection and police intervention, with courts and at times with the loss of important family members.

Individual psychotherapy

Individual psychotherapy is by no means always called for when a child has been sexually abused, but it can have something substantial to offer for children who have been left particularly bewildered and hurt by their experience. Themes such as anger, guilt, internal damage and dirt, secrecy and trust are likely to recur in any prolonged individual contact with an abused child, but it is perhaps the sexualization of experience and the issue of betrayal that most characterize the aftermath of sexual abuse. There may be particular problems around the establishment of a positive therapeutic rapport and also over the maintenance of appropriate boundaries; for these and other reasons good support for the therapy by concurrent work with the child's carers is very important.

There may also be a need for individual work with the child's non-abusing parent (usually the mother), particularly if memories of her own abuse have been raised by the abuse of the child, or if there are unresolved issues concerning separation from the abuser. Such work can also help move the adult to a position where she may be able to engage in dyadic therapy with her child (see below).

Dyadic therapy

Various combinations of dyadic therapy can be envisaged to meet the needs identified in the previous section. Joint work with the child and her or his non-abusing parent, or marital work with the non-abusing parents of a child sexually assaulted by a relative, friend or teacher are quite common combinations. Sometimes this work is preliminary to full family therapy, sometimes an adjunct to it; sometimes it may precede and sometimes follow individual therapy. In all instances the rationale is to provide a forum in which people severely affected by the abuse can share their feelings with each other, while offering the child protection from too much exposure to adult anger or despair.

Finally, there is a further general issue that arises from this quick listing of therapeutic options. Whatever work is undertaken with sexually abused children, it commonly places the professional in disturbing situations. Some of these are externally created: for example, knowing that one might have to testify in court and be cross-examined on the competence of one's work and judgement. Similarly, the sheer volume of work, with inter-agency consultation and report-writing, can be very daunting. Some of the pressures, however, arise from more internal sources. The difficulty of living with uncertainty was mentioned earlier; in addition, a wide range of feelings is commonly produced by exposure to the reality of sexual abuse: protectiveness towards the child, anger at the abuser, sexual arousal and curiosity, shame and embarrassment, bewilderment at what has been done and what allowed to occur. Dealing with these feelings is of major importance if the quality of professional work is to be high; acknowledging the reality of disturbing emotions, having a space to unwind and consult with colleagues, being properly supported by managers – these are crucial components of an appropriate response to child sexual abuse.

REFERENCES

Baker, A. and Duncan, S. (1985) Child sexual abuse: a study of prevalence in Great Britain, *Child Abuse and Neglect*, **9**, 457–67.
Bentovim, A. (1991) *Adolescent Abusers*, Unpublished paper, Tavistock Clinic, London.

146 *Child sexual abuse*

Bentovim, A., Elton, A., Hildebrand, J., Tranter, M. and Vizard, E. (1989) *Child Sexual Abuse Within the Family*, Wright, London.

Berliner, L. (1991) Treating the effects of child sexual abuse, in K. Murray and D. Gough (eds.) *Intervening in Child Sexual Abuse*, Scottish Academic Press, Glasgow.

Campbell, B. (1989) *Unofficial Secrets*, Virago, London.

Finkelhor, D. (1988) The trauma of child sexual abuse: Two models, in G. Wyatt and G. Powell (eds.) *Lasting Effects of Child Sexual Abuse*, Sage, London.

Finkelhor, D. (1991) The scope of the problem, in K. Murray and D. Gough (eds.) *Intervening in Child Sexual Abuse*, Scottish Academic Press, Glasgow.

Frosh, S. (1988) No man's land? The role of men working with sexually abused children, *British Journal of Guidance and Counselling*, 16, 1–10.

Glaser, D. (1992) Treatment issues in child sexual abuse, *British Journal of Psychiatry*, 159, 769-82.

Glaser, D. and Frosh, S. (1988) *Child Sexual Abuse*, Macmillan, London.

Haugaard, J. and Reppucci, N. (1988) *The Sexual Abuse of Children*, Jossey-Bass, San Francisco.

Herman, J. (1981) *Father-Daughter Incest*, Harvard University Press, Cambridge, MA.

Hildebrand, J. (1989) The use of groupwork in treating child sexual abuse, in A. Bentovim *et al. Child Sexual Abuse Within the Family*, Wright, London.

Jones, D. (1991) Interviewing children, in K. Murray and D. Gough (eds.) *Intervening in Child Sexual Abuse*, Scottish Academic Press, Glasgow.

Kidscape (1986) *Child Assault Prevention Programme*, Kidscape, London.

Levidow, L. (1989) Witches and seducers: Moral panics for our time, in B. Richards (ed.) *Crises of the Self*, Free Association Books, London.

MacLeod, M. and Sarraga, E. (1988) Challenging the orthodoxy: Towards a feminist theory and practice, *Feminist Review*, 28, 16–55.

Moore, K. (1991) *An Investigation into the Therapeutic Needs of Sexually Abused Children*, Unpublished PhD Thesis, University of London.

Mullen, P., Romans-Clarkson, S., Walton, V. and Herbison, G. (1988) Impact of sexual and physical abuse on women's mental health, *Lancet*, ii, 841–5.

Myers, J., Bays, J., Becker, J., Berliner, L., Corwin, D. and Saywitz, K. (1989) Expert testimony in child sexual abuse litigation, *Nebraska Law Review*, 68, 1.

Parton, N. (1985) *The Politics of Child Abuse*, Macmillan, London.

Pierce, L. and Pierce, R. (1987) Incestuous victimisation by juvenile sex offenders, *Journal of Family Violence* ,2, 351-64.

Russell, D. (1983) The incidence and prevalence of intrafamilial sexual abuse of female children, *Child Abuse and Neglect*, 7, 133–46.

Schechter, M. and Roberge, L. (1976) Child sexual abuse, in R. Helfer and C. Kempe (eds.) *Child Abuse and Neglect*, Ballinger, Cambridge, MA.

Section Three

Social Context

10

Counselling and social context

Jenny Bimrose

All counselling takes place within a social context. The relationship between this context and counselling has attracted little attention from theorists developing frameworks for practice over the past few decades. This is reflected in Britain by the low profile currently given to this aspect of counselling on training courses. There are, however, a steadily increasing number of writers in the area of counselling theory and practice who acknowledge the importance of the social context of counselling, and in some instances argue that issues related to context are central to the development of counselling theory and practice in the future (Ivey *et al.*, 1987).

As an outpatient myself recently, I saw the paramedic with responsibility for my treatment as a very young, attractive, energetic and capable woman, who had recently embarked on her professional career without ties such as children. During my twice-weekly treatment sessions, she spent time and effort establishing a counselling relationship with me. However, her suggestion for a daily exercise routine for me took no account of my particular social context as a middle-aged, full-time working mother of two small children. My explanations of why I was not making the progress expected were met with impatience and reproach. This reaction presumably stemmed from personal values held by my counsellor relating to the notion that my physical well-being should automatically take priority over everything else, together with an unrealistic view that it was possible for me to instruct my children to go and 'play quietly' in their rooms while I exercised for one hour three times a day!

All counsellors have, at some level, an awareness of and response to social context in their interactions with clients or patients. Egan and Cowan (1979), figuratively, present one such response:-

'The story goes that a person walking alongside a river sees someone drowning. This person jumps in, pulls the victim out, and begins artificial respiration. While this is going on, another person calls for help; the rescuer jumps into the water again and pulls the new victim out. This process re- peats itself several times until the rescuer gets up and walks away from the scene. A bystander approaches and asks in surprise where s/he is going, to which the rescuer replies, "I'm going upstream to find out who's pushing all these people in and see if I can stop it!" '

This story illustrates two closely related issues in respect of counselling practice. Firstly, whether counsellors should con- fine themselves to operating at the level of the individual, or contribute to changing the conditions that create the need in the patient or client for counselling. Secondly, whether counsellors should develop a more preventive role in their response to patients or clients; continue with what predominantly repre- sents 'crisis interventions'; or perhaps seek to develop a balance of the two approaches. The practitioner's view of these issues will be informed, in part at least, by their personal view of the relationship between counselling and the social context.

In this chapter, I will consider:-

- What is the social context?
- Three approaches to defining the social context:
  - Structural
  - Systems
  - Single Variable
- Three theoretical perspectives on social context:
  - Individualistic
  - Integrationist
  - Structuralist
- What are the implications for counselling?

DEFINING SOCIAL CONTEXT

The social context in which all counselling takes place is multidimensional, and each dimension (for example, individual, organizational and societal) will contain within it the potential for influencing the process of counselling. Both the counsellor and the patient/client bring to the counselling interactions their experiences of their own individual social contexts, and their views of the ability of this social context to accommodate development and/or change. These views may contrast sharply with and operate a powerful influence on the counselling interaction.

Additionally, most counselling takes place within the framework of an organization or institution which has the potential to influence both counselling process and outcome. For example, users of hospital services are defined as 'patients', and there exists, a whole set of normative behaviour patterns associated with the role of patients (such as the expectation that patients be the passive recipients of expert advice) which are likely to influence the way they approach a counselling session with a paramedic (Goffman, 1969). Equally, the setting in which a counsellor is working may be poorly resourced materially, and this is likely to affect the counselling process and outcome in a number of ways (perhaps even at the basic level of the number of sessions offered).

A further dimension is the wider society in which the counsellor and client, and the 'host' organization or institution, are located. The dominant systems of beliefs, or ideologies, operating within the wider society have the potential to impact in a powerful way on counselling practice. One unambiguous example of what is meant by this is contained in the transcript of an interview of the Head of the Counselling and Careers Unit at the University of Witwatersrand, Johannesburg, South Africa, conducted in August 1989, which explores issues arising from counselling under a system of apartheid (Dryden, 1990). At one point in the interview, Andrew Swart (the Head of the Unit) discusses pressures arising from counselling interactions with clients. He expresses his belief that counsellors in South Africa see a significant number of clients who have been traumatized by South African society, and quotes the following example:

'A student who had been apparently randomly detained by the security police comes to mind. This person had not been politically active and had been deliberately avoiding political activity. However, due to unexplained circumstances which occurred during a security police raid, he was detained for 60 days in solitary confinement; and after he was released he came for counselling. I was confronted with a sense of outrage and the trauma that this person had been subjected to. This put pressure on me, because what should I, as a professional, do about something that is so blatantly unjust? Do I just treat the person and help him to work through his feelings of outrage and encourage him (or her) to cope more or less normally, or do I take the matter further? It raises uncomfortable questions of professional ethics and personal interest.'

(Dryden, 1990, p. 309)

This represents an extreme example of a client seeking counselling help as a direct consequence of the dominant ideology of apartheid operating in the wider social context. However, counsellors in British (or any other) society do find themselves in situations not totally dissimilar when confronted with patients or clients who have been the victims of actual or symbolic violence, such as rape victims or victims of racial abuse or attack.

THREE APPROACHES TO DEFINING THE SOCIAL CONTEXT

Several writers from various theoretical persuasions, contributing to the development of counselling theory and practice over several decades, have mentioned the importance of the social context. A smaller number of writers have argued that social context is of central importance. Given, it is claimed, that well in excess of 250 theories of counselling and therapy currently exist (Ivey *et al.*, 1987), it is perhaps hardly surprising that there is little consensus on which dimensions of the social context have primary significance, or in what way. It is, however, possible to identify three broad tendencies. Firstly, there are those who argue the all-pervasive importance of social *structures* to counselling and psychotherapy; secondly, there is a *systems* approach to context; thirdly, there is increasing interest in developing approaches that represent consideration of *single variables* of context, notably race and gender.

Structural approach

Social context can be conceptualized in terms of the structures which define the relationships between individuals and groups. Smail (1987, 1991) identifies power as over-ridingly important, as it defines the culture, ideology and class of an individual. These, in turn, define many 'environmental' experiences, such as those determined by school, work, housing, etc. Woolfe (1983) argues that counselling be viewed as a 'social enterprise' which takes full account of the social, economic and political structures within society. Ivey *et al.* (1987), in developing an integrated model of skills, theory and practice for counselling and psychotherapy, identify culture as the missing dimension from the majority of helping theories, and imply that an awareness of issues arising from an individual's age, race, gender, socio-economic status and religious background is of critical importance to any counsellor's professional effectiveness.

Although the use of key concepts amongst such writers differs, they all refer to those structures within society producing and/or maintaining inequality among individuals and/or groups. It is these inequalities that play an important part in influencing an individual's life chances and, arguably, their potential for self-development. The examples they quote represent a new trend stressing the importance of social structure to counselling. These writers use terminology normally associated with the academic discipline of sociology, but without applying the associated rigour in their use. Failure to acknowledge the difficulties encountered by attempts to arrive at acceptable definitions of such terms may result in misunderstanding and confusion amongst the readers whose views these writers seek to influence.

Systems approach

In contrast, Egan and Cowan (1979) provide a detailed 'systems model' of social context. Based on a 'developmental' approach to counselling, they argue that it is essential for individuals to achieve an understanding of the social settings in which human development takes place. A better understanding of how they are being affected by the systems in their lives will enable individuals to be better equipped to 'cope with, co-operate with, and challenge these systems' (Egan and Cowan, 1979).

Their categorization of systems is presented as operating at four levels:

1. *Microsystem* – small, immediate systems of everyday lives, e.g. family, friendship groups, immediate work settings and classrooms;
2. *Mesosystem* – the network of personal settings and the interactions among them, e.g. events at work can affect people at home, friends, other people at school;
3. *Exosystem* – larger institutions within society that indirectly influence personal systems and networks of personal settings, e.g. governmental agencies, the economic system, the media and religious organizations;
4. *Macrosystem* – refers to the culture that shapes individuals, organizations and institutions, pervading all aspects of life.

One of the goals for counselling, then, becomes to equip people with a working knowledge of these social systems that will enable them to enhance their own development in the social context in which they operate. Referring to my earlier personal example (p.149), a goal for that counselling relationship would have been for the paramedic to explore with me the constraints of my immediate situation (microsystem) before exploring the possibility of my extended family and friends (mesosystem) and work environment (exosystem) providing the support necessary for me to undertake a negotiated and realistic exercise programme.

Single variable approaches

Focusing on a single social variable, such as race or gender, is another emergent trend emphasizing the importance of context to counselling. Identifying a concern that the theories underpinning most counselling practice have developed from white, male, middle-class orientations, such writers question the legitimacy of using these theories for counselling clients from different backgrounds, such as those from different racial backgrounds and clients of a different gender (Sue, 1981; Chaplin, 1988). In so doing, these writers are beginning to identify issues related to the common characteristic defining their chosen client group, and the implications arising from those issues for life chances and therefore for counselling practice.

In my earlier personal example, my gender, my motherhood, and my being employed together limited the possible outcomes of counselling in a way that the counsellor did not acknowledge.

THREE THEORETICAL PERSPECTIVES ON SOCIAL CONTEXT

The theoretical perspectives on which counselling practice is based are numerous and complex, as are the definitions of counselling itself. Ivey *et al.* (1987) liken the task of achieving an understanding of this range of competing views of the world to finding a way through a maze. However confusing the complexity of theory and practice may be, the debate which gives rise to these competing views is essential to a rigorous and continued development of this area. The same principle applies to the development of perspectives on the social context of counselling. A threefold categorization of different perspectives contributing to understanding of social context is offered next as one possible method of introducing coherence to an understanding of this area. These are 'individualistic', 'integrationist' and 'structuralist'.

Individualistic

Counselling originates from the academic discipline of psychology, and has used mainstream psychological theories as the basis for the development of a range of practices and therapies for use with clients. In seeking to increase understanding of various aspects of human behaviour, psychology starts at the level of the individual (though it should be acknowledged that within psychology there are separate schools of thought that differ in their view of the centrality of the individual). As a result, therefore, of deriving from this particular academic tradition, counselling theory locates explanations relating to the client's need for help within the individual. In so doing, these theories separate an individual's need for help, however this is manifested, from their social context, and thus define social context as irrelevant to the counselling process.

An example of one such theory that has been of particular importance to the development of counselling practice is Rogers' (1957, 1961) person-centred approach. Deriving from the existential-humanistic tradition, one of Rogers' central ideas is that individuals are able to determine their own destinies. Thus, control lies within the individual, rather than externally in the social context.

Another influence on the development of counselling is the psychodynamic school and in particular its concept of the 'unconscious'. In this approach individuals are unaware of what is motivating them towards action, and it is conflict arising from the past, rather than the social context of the present, which creates personal crises requiring the need for 'therapy' for the 'patient'.

Integrationist

Egan's 'systems model' (p. 153) is an example of an attempt to integrate an understanding of social context in an approach to counselling practice. The model developed for use by Egan and Cowan (1979) for counselling practitioners is based on Lewin's (1935) equation:

$$B = f(P \times E)$$

where behaviour (**B**) is a function of the interaction between person (**P**) and environment (**E**). Egan develops this equation to provide one incorporating the concept of 'system':

$$HD = f[(P \leftrightarrow S) \times (S \leftrightarrow S)]$$

In this equation, human development (**HD**) is a function of the interaction between people (**P**) and the human systems (**S**) in which they are involved, and of the interaction of these systems with each other. The following propositions regarding human development throughout life indicate the meaning of this term used in the model:

- Biological development assumes a critical role, particularly during certain life stages.
- Human development is age-related but not age-specific.
- Human development is bound up in the human systems of our lives.

- Working knowledge and skills for living are essential to human development through life.
- Human support is a crucial resource for the developing person in any life stage.
- The meaning of the word 'development' varies with the cultural context.

(Egan and Cowan, 1979)

In addition to presenting a detailed account of four levels of the human systems in which this development occurs (see p. 154), a process model for implementing the systems model is outlined, the basic steps of which are:

- diagnosis
- goal setting
- programme development
- implementation and evaluation

(Egan and Cowan, 1979)

These two models (systems and process), together with definitions of human development and systems, are complemented by an account of those skills needed to implement this approach to counselling:

- **Skills relating to physical development**
  - the skills of physical fitness
  - the skills of personal health care
  - athletic skills
  - aesthetic use of the body
  - grooming

- **Skills relating to intellectual development**
  - the ability to translate knowledge into working knowledge
  - learning how to learn

- **Self-management skills**
  - the ability to use a working theory of personality
  - the ability to apply the basic principles of behaviour to practical situations
  - problem-solving and programme-development skills

- **Value-clarification skills**

- **Skills of interpersonal involvement**
  - self-presentation skills
  - responding skills
  - skills of challenging others

- **Skills of small-group involvement**
  - clarifying the goals of the group
  - initiating in a group
  - using the resources of a group
  - participating effectively in a group

(Egan and Cowan, 1979)

This represents a comprehensive, if formidable, skills training requirement. Overall,this example of an integrated approach considers the nature of the relationship between individuals and their social context, how this may be positively influenced within a counselling framework, and additionally provides an account of the skills training requirement for its implementation.

Sue (1981) provides another example of what may be categorized an 'integrationist' approach to social context. Focusing, as he does, on the single contextual variable of cultural difference, Sue presents 'an integrated conceptual framework by which to view how cross-cultural counselling relates to wider social forces, the counsellor–client relationship, and the culturally different in the United States'. This is motivated by what Sue defines as a disturbing absence of texts which could be used in training to enhance the counselling services offered to clients from ethnic minority backgrounds. This situation continues to exist despite an increasing weight of criticism levelled against current counselling practice 'as being demeaning, irrelevant and oppressive toward the culturally different'.

Issues relating to cross-cultural counselling are explored around a series of questions posed:

- What is cross-cultural counselling?
- Is it any different from other forms of counselling?
- Do we really need to view minority clients as being different from anyone else?
- How can counselling be accused of being a form of cultural oppression?
- Why do minority clients distrust counselling so much?

- Can a person of another race/culture counsel a client effectively?
- What are some of the barriers to effective cross-cultural counselling?
- How may they be overcome?

(Sue, 1981)

A careful consideration of such important and contentious issues becomes part of the process of adopting an integrated model for cross-cultural counselling. The result is the identification of the characteristics of the 'culturally skilled counsellor', divided into three categories of competences:

1. **Awareness of assumptions, values and biases**
   A culturally skilled counsellor
   - has moved to being culturally aware and valuing and respecting differences
   - is aware of own values and biases, and how they may affect clients
   - is comfortable with the differences that exist between counsellor and client
   - is sensitive to circumstances which may dictate referral of client to a member of own culture
   - acknowledges and is aware of own racist attitudes, beliefs and feelings

2. **Understanding the world view of the culturally different client**
   A culturally skilled counsellor
   - possesses specific knowledge and information about the particular client(s) he/she is working with
   - has a good understanding of the sociopolitical system re inequality
   - has a clear and explicit knowledge and understanding of the generic characteristics of counselling and therapy
   - is aware of institutional barriers which prevent clients from using services, etc.

3. **Development of appropriate intervention strategies and techniques**
   A culturally skilled counsellor is
   - able to generate a wide variety of verbal and non-verbal responses

- able to send and receive verbal and non-verbal messages accurately and 'appropriately'
- able to exercise institutional intervention skills on behalf of client when necessary
- aware of his/her helping style, recognizesthe limitations he/she possesses, and can anticipate the impact upon the culturally different client

(Sue and Sue, 1990)

It is only those counsellors who can demonstrate competence in all of these areas who can be regarded as culturally skilled.

Structuralist

Proponents of what is labelled here as a 'structuralist approach' to social context derive predominantly from the professional background of psychotherapy. Agreement about boundaries between counselling and psychotherapy is yet to be achieved, and both terms include complex variations. Nonetheless, the contributions of these psychotherapists to our understanding of the role of social context continues to be of significance for both counselling practice and therapy.

The approach has developed from a deep dissatisfaction with the academic roots of psychotherapy, embedded as they are in the Freudian tradition of psychoanalysis. Smail (1987, 1991) argues that psychology in general, and psychoanalysis in particular, is seriously flawed because it fails to incorporate any consideration of social context in its academic framework, and this failure translates to the practice of therapy. Smail argues that the strivings of psychologists towards scientific objectivism have resulted in the production of a body of theory which is now used to manipulate and exploit individuals. Therapy is an example of how this occurs, since it has established itself as a 'treatment' for 'patients' – the implication being that it is possible to 'cure' human distress at an individual level. The assumption underlying this whole process is that human distress originates at the level of the individual. Thus, psychotherapy becomes a 'magical' cure for individual illness, and therapists are able to avoid considering that the human distress therapy seeks to cure is actually caused by damage individuals do to each other within the constraints and influences of wider social structures. Smail's criticism of psychotherapy extends to the claim that it is vested interest that prevents, acknowledgement of the real causes of human distress, since if the profession admitted that human distress is caused by the operation of power structures within society, the need for therapy would, effectively, no longer exist. Psychology, he argues, is used to mystify our understanding of reasons for individual behaviour, and therapy is used to 'stifle anguished protests'.

This perspective thus develops the notion that therapy and counselling are methods of social control, seeking to contain any potential protests that might result in fundamental structural change. Smail presents an analysis of British society in the 1980s as driven by materialism. The dominant political ideology of this decade has permitted indifference and greed to predominate, defining money as the prime motivating force and encouraging the mindless searching for pleasure in the form of material acquisition, without any regard for human suffering or for damage done to animals and the environment as a consequence.

Woolfe (1983) agrees with much of Smail's analysis, though his view of the primary cause of the failure of counselling to take any account of context rests, less contentiously, with the emphasis given in training to the amount of choice exercised by individuals and to person-centredness, rather than with the whole academic tradition of psychology. His focus is similarly the issue of social control:

'The question to be asked becomes one of whether counsellors are part of the solution or part of the problem.'

(Woolfe, 1983)

He does, however, emerge as a defender of core aspects of the counselling process as potentially constructive, arguing that outdated concepts such as 'self-actualization' and 'fully functioning person' – themselves products of a 1960s Californian social context – need fundamental updating to take account of the current crises of poverty, unemployment and various social and racial conflicts.

This structural perspective, implicating as it does changes in the social structures in which counselling takes place, is an uncomfortable view with which to engage. It does, however, deserve a response. As Pilgrim (1991) claims:

'The self-doubts of radical professionals have triggered a debate about psychotherapy and its social blinkers which is likely to continue to be a permanent challenge to their conservative colleagues.'

IMPLICATIONS FOR COUNSELLING PRACTICE

Increasing attention is being paid to the relationship between social context and counselling practice. This is a compelling reason for practitioners, trainers and students of counselling to become familiar with the different dimensions of the debate, so that they can, at the very least, identify the perspective from which they are themselves operating (or intend to operate) in the future.

The practical implications for counselling practice will vary according to which of the perspectives is adopted by the practitioner. To illustrate this point, the practical implications for practice of each of the three perspectives identified above will now be briefly considered.

Individualistic

Practitioners who retain the belief that their clients will be best served by the traditional theoretical perspectives derived from psychology will have no need to make any change to their counselling practice. So, for example, those operating within a Rogerian, person-centred framework will continue to believe that counsellors need no special skills or knowledge to respond to any client they seek to help. The core skills of empathy, acceptance and understanding are all the counsellor needs to establish the quality of relationship essential for the helping process.

Integrationist

In contrast to this, practitioners operating from an integrationist viewpoint will require considerable training input initially, so that they acquire the knowledge base needed, together with the development of the necessary skills. Their practice of counselling will involve counsellors 'giving away' (Egan and Cowan, 1979) their skills (e.g. assertiveness training) in group sessions so that these skills, needed to change systems, may be more efficiently cascaded throughout the community.

Additionally, it may involve counsellors working with groups of clients (e.g. rape victims, unemployed clients) to enable them to understand the social structures that have caused the need for them to seek counselling help. It may also require the counsellor to become involved themselves in changing the system on behalf of their clients. These ways of working will complement individual counselling, during which counsellors will operate with a high level of awareness of social context.

Structuralist

Implications emerging from this perspective are more abstract, and therefore seemingly less attainable for students and practitioners. At one level, there exists the requirement for the development of a different theoretical base on which practice may be based. Smail (1991) advocates the development of an 'environmentalist psychology' as a more appropriate theoretical basis for working with individuals in distress. At another level, this approach implicates a fundamental restructuring of society and its dominant values, so that individuals are more inclined to care for and support each other, thus reducing the need for specialist help. Related to this somewhat utopian notion of engendering a more caring attitude within society is the requirement for therapists to empower patients to help themselves by changing the social systems damaging them. Indeed, perhaps part of the threat or challenge of this particular perspective is that it is difficult for the individual counsellor to identify an appropriate, and achievable, response.

CONCLUSION

Social context has remained essentially the invisible issue in relation to counselling theory, training and practice over the past few decades. Despite the contributions of writers such as Egan and Cowan (1979), Sue (1981) and Sue and Sue (1990) providing frameworks for training and practice, contributions remain very small in number. They tend to involve resource implications for training and practice, so perhaps it is not surprising that their impact has been marginal. Radical contributions, such as those from Smail (1987, 1991) and Woolfe (1983), are also relatively small in number, somewhat abstract in the concepts they present, and have been the subject of some curiosity, ridicule and heated debate. They have not, however, so far provided the stimulus for radical change.

It seems those writers concerning themselves with single contextual variables such as race or gender are the most likely to change attitudes towards the importance of social context to counselling practice. Perhaps this is attributable to the higher profile equal opportunities legislation has given to racial and gender differences and their social consequences. Whatever the reason, it seems that students, trainers and practitioners alike are finding it increasingly difficult to ignore the possibility that clients of a different racial background or gender pose a particular challenge in terms of their deriving a satisfactory outcome from the counselling relationship.

It seems certain that in the development of counselling, wider issues related to social context will continue to be considered. Increasingly, there is pressure on training courses in counselling to offer an input on social context. If this succeeds in increasing the level of debate by raising levels of awareness, the quality of counselling practice, in the longer term, can only be enhanced.

REFERENCES

Chaplin, J. (1988) *Feminist Counselling in Action*, Sage, London.

Dryden, W. (1990) Counselling under apartheid: an interview with Andrew Swart, *British Journal of Guidance and Counselling*, **18**, no.3, 308–20.

Egan, G. and Cowan, R.M. (1979) *People and Systems: An integrative approach to human development*, Brooks/Cole, California.

Goffman, E. (1969) *The Presentation of Self in Everyday Life*, Allen Lane, London.

Ivey, A.E., Ivey, M.B. and Simek-Downing, L. (1987) *Counselling and Psychotherapy: Integrating skills, theory and practice*, Prentice-Hall, London.

Lewin, K. (1935) *A Dynamic Theory of Personality*, McGraw Hill, New York.

Pilgrim, D. (1991) Psychotherapy and social blinkers, *The Psychologist*, **2**, 52–5.

Rogers, C. (1957) The necessary and sufficient conditions of therapeutic personality change, *Journal of Consulting Psychology*, **21**, 95–103.

Rogers, C. (1961) *On Becoming A Person*, Houghton Mifflin, Boston.

Smail, D. (1987) *Taking Care: An alternative to therapy*, Dent, London.

Smail, D. (1991) Towards a radical environmentalist psychology of help, *The Psychologist*, **2**, 61–5.

Sue, D.W. (1981) *Counselling the Culturally Different: Theory and practice*, Wiley, New York.

Sue, D.W. and Sue, D. (1990) *Counselling the Culturally Different: Theory and practice*, 2nd edn, Wiley, New York.

Woolfe, R. (1983) Counselling in a world of crisis: Towards a sociology of counselling, *International Journal of Advanced Counselling*, **6**, 167–76.

11

Psychopathology: classification, aetiological theories and treatments

Jane Ussher

Psychopathology is an emotive term. It connotes derangement, disturbance and an absence of control. It is not a term which we would readily apply to ourselves, determined to assert our normality, our sanity. Yet every year thousands of individuals will be diagnosed, classified and treated for psychological problems, because they are deemed to be suffering from a form of psychopathology, or what we might colloquially term madness. These individuals are not strange or abhorrent, as the imagination might portray them; they are ordinary people. But the taboo and stigma still associated with madness in the late twentieth century often results in their suffering in silence. This is a silence that needs to be broken.

In the late twentieth century, highly organized mental health professions have evolved in order to provide explanations and treatments for madness. These include psychiatry, clinical psychology, social work, counselling, psychiatric nursing and those practising a range of different therapies. Whilst historically only the most extreme cases of aberrant behaviour or the most violent distress might have come under the umbrella of the experts, today a whole gamut of psychological problems, ranging from mild distress to full-blown psychosis, can be diagnosed, classified and pronounced open to cure.

Yet the classification, analysis and treatment of psychopathology is not as straightforward as might first appear. There is much controversy and disagreement over the notion of what psychopathology is. The very term implies a deviation from the norm, which is always culturally and historically specific. So what is deemed mad in Western industrialized society, such as the hearing of voices, which indicates a diagnosis of schizophrenia, may be deemed divine inspiration or connection with the gods in a different culture.

There is also disagreement over this notion of madness as illness which pervades the mental health professions of today, as this is seen to imply a reductionist aetiology. There is disagreement over the cause of problems, and their appropriate cure, with challenges to the legitimacy of the continued supremacy of the psychiatric profession underlying many of these critiques. Yet despite the healthy scepticism meted out to many of the current experts in the field of madness, the reality of the misery and distress experienced by many individuals who come forward for treatment cannot be denied, and therefore their difficulties need to be taken seriously and appropriate help offered, if at all possible.

In order to provide an insight into the many different theories and therapies currently available, and the different notions of what psychopathology actually is, this chapter will examine the current classification of behaviour and symptoms considered to be evidence of psychopathology, the competing aetiological explanations offered by psychiatry, psychology and the sociocultural critics, and the implications of these different approaches for individual assessment and care.

THE HISTORY OF MADNESS

One of the important strands of any explanation of our current understanding of psychopathology is the historical perspective. Madness, now deemed mental illness, may be framed within a scientific prism in the late twentieth century, safely contained within taxonomic paradigms which legitimize the authority of psychiatrists and clinical psychologists, but this has not always been the case. Prior to what has been termed 'the age of enlightenment' (Foucault, 1967) in the late eighteenth century, aberrant behaviour was construed and controlled within a theological framework, the clergy providing an explanation for deviancy and distress. Those who might now be termed ill were often viewed as infected with an evil spirit, perhaps 'shot' into them by a witch. Women who heard voices were not defined as ill, as schizophrenic, but as saints hearing the voice of God. The mad were also conceived of as animal-like, as almost bestial, a belief which sanctioned harsh treatment and punishment, or physical neglect in the notorious asylums, as was described by La Salpetriere at the end of the eighteenth century:

> 'Madwomen seized with fits of violence are chained like dogs at their cell doors, and separated from keepers and visitors alike by a long corridor protected by an iron grille; through this grille is passed their food and the straw on which they sleep; by means of rakes, part of the filth that surrounds them is cleaned out.'
>
> (Foucault, 1967, p. 72)

These conditions may seem barbaric today and a far cry from the notion of therapy or care, but as Scull (1979, p.64) argued, 'the resort to fear, force and coercion (was) a tactic entirely appropriate to the management of brutes!'. The notion of madness as illness was not current prior to the nineteenth century, as madness was construed as a disorder of control, the absence of reason, or a malevolent force (Foucault, 1967). Yet in the late eighteenth century the lay asylum keepers who housed and controlled both the insane and a whole range of societal outcasts were usurped by a new grouping of experts, the medically trained psychiatrists. Porter (1987, p.166) has described them as the 'medical entrepreneurs' who heralded in the new 'age of reason' and asserted that madness was illness with a clear somatic basis, with the predominant theory being that the brain was at fault. They established the premise that care, rather than punishment or incarceration, was the appropriate response, and maintained that science was the force which would provide the framework necessary for adequate explanation and cure. As the English psychiatrist Henry Maudsely claimed in 1873:

> 'The observation and classification of mental disorders have been so exclusively psychological that we have not sincerely realized the fact that they illustrate the same pathological principles as other diseases, are produced in the same way, and must be investigated in the same spirit of positive research.'
>
> (Baruch and Treacher, 1978, p. 35)

It was this nineteenth century emphasis on the scientific validity of the psychiatric control over madness that paved the way for the dominant discourse of today, that which clearly and concisely defines psychopathology within a positivistic framework, where symptoms are grouped together as part of syndromes and the process of clear classification is a central part of our current understanding of psychopathology.

TAXONOMY AND CLASSIFICATION

The classification system of the German psychiatrist Kraepelin, first published in 1883, provided the foundation for the taxonomic analysis of syndromes and symptoms utilized by a majority of mental health professionals today. This adoption of standard psychiatric labels and descriptions was established in order to allow comparison of research data and treatments across patients, and to facilitate the development of standardized assessments and interventions. However, it also had the function of legitimizing the authority of the medically trained psychiatrists in this arena, and served to reify the symptoms as recognizable entities or illnesses.

Within this taxonomic framework, disparate symptoms have been systematically organized into a collection of distinct and discrete syndromes, which are isolated and considered as independent entities. The resultant categories are now established within the bibles of psychiatry, devised by the American Psychiatric Association or the World Health Organization: the DSM 111R (Diagnostic and Statistical Manual of Mental Disorders) and the ICD-9 (International Classification of Diseases). Madness is now more clinically described as 'mental disorder', and distinguished thus:

'A clinically significant behavioural or psychological syndrome or pattern that occurs in an individual and that is typically either associated with either a painful symptom (distress) or impairment in one or more important areas of functioning (disability). In addition, there is an inference that there is a behavioural, psychological or biological dysfunction, and that the disturbance is not only in the relationship between the individual and society.'

(ICD-9)

In order to illustrate the range of symptoms and behaviours encapsulated by this diagnostic framework, it will be useful to examine the DSM IIIR, which divides mental disorder into a number of different 'axes', the first two being the means of classifying 'abnormal behaviour'. As is evident from the list below, a whole range of psychiatric categories exist in order to encompass long term and short term, major and minor difficulties.

Axis I

* *Disorders usually first evident in infancy, childhood or adolescence* (mental retardation, attention deficit disorder, conduct disorder, anxiety disorders of childhood or adolescence, other disorders of infancy, childhood or adolescence, eating disorders, stereotyped movement disorders, other disorders with physical manifestations, pervasive developmental disorders)
* *Organic mental disorders* (dementia, delirium, amnesic syndrome, organic delusional syndrome, organic hallucinations, organic mood syndrome, organic anxiety syndrome, organic personality syndrome)
* *Psycho-active substance use disorders* (including alcohol, barbiturate, amphetamine, tobacco and cannabis abuse)
* *Schizophrenic disorders* (disorganized, catatonic, paranoid, undifferentiated, residual)
* *Delusional (paranoid) disorders*
* *Neurotic disorders*
* *Affective (mood) disorders* (bipolar disorder, major depression, other specific affective disorder, atypical affective disorder)
* *Anxiety disorders* (phobias, obsessive compulsive disorder, panic disorder, generalized anxiety, post traumatic stress disorder)
* *Somatoform disorders* (conversion disorder, psychogenic pain disorder, hypochondrias, atypical somatoform disorder)
* *Dissociative disorders* (psychogenic amnesia, psychogenic fugue, multiple personality, depersonalization disorder)
* *Sexual disorders* (gender identity disorders, paraphilias – i.e. fetishism, transvestism, paedophilia, sexual masochism/sadism – psychosexual dysfunctions – i.e. inhibited sexual desire/excitement, inhibited orgasm, premature ejaculation, vaginismus)

- *Sleep disorders*
- *Psychological factors affecting physical condition*

Axis II

- *Personality disorders* (paranoid, schizotypal, histrionic, narcissistic, antisocial, borderline, avoidant, dependant, obsessive-compulsive, passive-aggressive)
- *Developmental disorders* (academic skills disorders, language and speech disorders, mental retardation, pervasive developmental disorder)

In order to illustrate how these diagnoses might be applied, a number of brief case descriptions are provided below, illustrating some of the very different manifestations of symptoms which may be experienced by individuals. Each of these individuals was suffering serious disruption to life because of their problems, and would be likely to receive psychiatric or psychological help, were it available.

Deborah, aged 24, diagnosed as suffering from agoraphobia (anxiety disorder)

Deborah was trained as a nurse, and had had a very successful career until she was involved in a car crash where her best friend was seriously injured. Following the crash Deborah felt continuously agitated and was not able to go near a car, because feelings of panic would overcome her. Her symptoms included increased heart rate, rapid breathing, sweating hands, shaking and a sensation of dizziness. Her thoughts contained uncontrollable fears that something terrible would happen to her. Over a number of months she found that she experienced the panic more and more frequently when she was out, and only when she was safely at home did she feel in control. She started to avoid going out on her own, and then found that even when she thought about leaving the house she would feel sensations of panic. She eventually had to resign from her job because she couldn't face going out at all. She was now completely confined to the house.

Simon, aged 40, diagnosed as paranoid schizophrenic

Simon lived with his elderly parents and worked as a clerk

in a local bank. He had always been a loner but had started to appear increasingly strange to his colleagues, who noticed that he was very secretive about his work, and more withdrawn on social occasions. Simon was convinced that there was a plot to ruin him, and that espionage was involved. He believed that his phone was tapped and that if he didn't follow certain rituals at work, people would be able to read his thoughts. He looked for evidence for his fears all of the time, and invariably found confirmation. He coped at work for some time, but was sent for psychiatric assessment when his parents noticed that he was barricading himself into his bedroom at night, so that no-one could get at him. At the hospital he was convinced that the doctors were involved in the conspiracy, and thus he was adamant that he was not going to be fooled by the plot to incarcerate him, so he refused to speak.

Joan, aged 38, diagnosed as depressed

Joan was a mother of three children, who spent much of her day looking after the house and caring for her children's needs.

However, she was finding life increasingly difficult and was filled with an overwhelming desire to run away, or end her life. She felt worthless and unhappy, not being able to see any reason for continuing with life. She had no appetite and had lost 20 pounds in weight over the last six months. Her sleep patterns were disrupted, as she woke up very early in the morning, having had great difficulty sleeping all night. During the day she felt continuously tired and everything she did was a great effort.

This may at first glance appear very clearcut – the classification systems providing a comprehensive description of a range of different problems and difficulties an individual may experience, which can be identified as part of a particular syndrome by a professional, usually a psychiatrist. Following diagnosis, appropriate treatment can be applied in an effective manner, in these three examples, for anxiety, schizophrenia and depression. However, it is not that simple.

PARADIGMS AND THEORIES

The decision about what type of intervention, if any, will be offered, and the explanation offered of the aetiology of psycho-pathology will be dependent upon the paradigm adopted by the mental health professional who is approached, as is illustrated below. For there is no one agreed analysis of madness, and no agreement about the appropriate response.

Biological theories

The traditional 'medical model', which reduces psychopathology to physical aetiology, has been transformed from crude analogies between the various 'humours' and madness to a sophisticated array of theories attesting to the biochemical basis of symptomatology. Currently dominating psychiatric thinking and therapies, the biological approach invariably assumes a genetic basis for psychopathology, exemplified by the comment, 'Depression runs in families. Children who receive the depressive gene or genes become vulnerable, or predisposed, to affective disorder' (Gold, 1986). The whole range of psychiatric syndromes, including anxiety, alcoholism, schizophrenia, depression and personality disorders, have been attributed to organic or genetic factors. Malfunctions in the brain or deficiencies in circulating hormones have been posited as the underlying cause, clearly leading to physical treatments and therapies.

The use of physical treatments in the context of psychiatric hospitalization has a long history. From the physical incarceration of the early asylums, the leeching, enforced bed rest, or the crude electrical treatment of the nineteenth century, the belief in the efficacy of a bodily cure was an intrinsic part of the medical response to madness. Three of the treatments most commonly used in the early part of the twentieth century were insulin shock, where the patient was loaded with insulin until a coma ensued, electroconvulsive therapy (ECT), where electric shocks were sent through the brain, usually under anaesthetic, and lobotomy, less frequently used but most clearly demonstrating the reductionist viewpoint, as the offending organ, part of the diseased brain, is literally removed.

Whilst ECT is still advocated for a wide range of problems, including depression (and particularly puerperal depression), schizophrenia and mania, pharmacological treatments have become the dominant form of intervention. Psychiatric hospitalization is no longer common, as the policy of 'care in the community' has resulted in the widespread closure of long-stay hospitals, with a concomitant emphasis on pharmacological control. For whilst today's psychiatrists undoubtedly do use psychological therapies, these are invariably seen as supplements to the drug treatments. These include tricyclic antidepressants (such as amitriptyline and imipramine) and monoamine oxidase inhibitors (such as phenelzine and tranylcypromine) for depression; for anxiety, tranquillizers (such as benzodiazepines), sedatives or lithium; and for psychosis, the antipsychotic phenothiazines. Thus if referred to a psychiatrist, Joan, Simon and Deborah would have been likely to receive a physical diagnosis and pharmacological treatment for their distress.

Yet physical treatments are not the only solution open to mental health professionals, for a number of different psychological and social theories have evolved over the last 50 years. In addition, the physical treatments have been criticized, ECT for causing serious memory loss and for being based on coercion rather than cure, and drug treatments for being based on faulty theorizing or for being the cause of many iatrogenic illnesses – symptoms *caused* by the drugs, which may be worse than the original symptoms which the psychiatrists set out to cure. The psychological therapies thus attempt to provide explanation and intervention within a less invasive sphere, and to acknowledge the psychological roots of distress.

Psychoanalysis

The first recognized 'talking cure' was psychoanalysis, based on the work of Sigmund Freud (1856 – 1939). At the foundation of psychoanalysis is the assumption that unconscious desires and fears underlie and motivate behaviour, and that childhood experiences often lead to adult neurosis. Freud argued that the constant battle for dominance between parts of the unconscious mind (the ego, id and superego) resulted in the neurotic anxiety which he deemed to be at the root of the majority of psychological disturbances, and in the blockage or repression of unconscious impulses. Successful resolution of the stages of psychosexual development, the oral, anal, phallic and genital stages, leads to psychological health; unsuccessful resolution, accompanied by introjection and repression, leads to neurosis – to madness. Within this framework, Joan's depression (above) could have been seen as resulting from loss in childhood or unconscious conflicts, to be resolved in psychoanalytic therapy.

Psychoanalytic therapy creates an alliance between the therapist and the healthy part of the patient's ego, in order to resolve the unconscious conflicts which lead to neurosis. The patient is allowed to resolve the earlier conflicts which are at the root of distress through facing the repressed feelings in the safety of the analytic setting, and moving towards resolution in the light of adult reality. If the repression is no longer in operation, the ego should be able to develop normally. Classic psychoanalysis employs the use of free association, dream analysis and interpretation to allow the patient to express unresolved conflict and to loosen defence mechanisms. Much of the emphasis in the treatment is on the therapeutic relationship and particularly on the 'transference', the feelings directed towards the therapist in the analytic sessions which are actually feelings for significant figures in the patient's past. The interpretation of these feelings, such as anger at the analyst being interpreted as anger at rejection by a parent, can allow the patient to realize her repressed feelings and, through expressing them, resolve them. In recent years, short term 'psychodynamic therapy' has evolved, wherein the basic premise of resolution of unconscious desires is adhered to, but the intervention is more focused and of a shorter duration (Malan, 1979; Casement, 1985).

Behaviour therapy: learning and reinforcement

During the 1950s, one of the paradigms which evolved as a rival to psychoanalysis was behavioural theory and therapy. Behaviourism does not concentrate on the unconscious but on observable behaviour and the environment, arguing that all behaviour is learnt and that psychopathology is either a result of faulty learning or of problems in the environment. Within this view, Deborah's anxiety could be seen to result from the traumatic event of the crash, resulting in a fear associated with cars and avoidance of the outside world because of its association with her previous distress; an anxiety which does not reduce because of her avoidance.

Behaviour therapy has been used most extensively with anxiety, phobias and depression. One of the most commonly used interventions is 'systematic desensitization', where learned associations are seen as being the cause of anxiety and treatment involves gradual exposure to the feared object or situation, resulting in the experience of the anxiety as non-threatening, which thus then reduces anxiety. So a person who is diagnosed as agoraphobic, such as Deborah, would be taught to relax and then encouraged to venture out of the house in a number of graduated stages, so that she could learn that what she feared, the outside world, was not threatening. Other behavioural techniques such as modelling, role playing or assertiveness training are also used to change people's behaviour, and thus reduce psychological symptoms.

Cognitive theories

Over the last 20 years psychologists have recognized that learning alone cannot account for psychopathology. This has led to the development of cognitive theories and therapies, where thoughts, beliefs, attitudes and memories are seen as factors underlying behaviour. Depression (Beck and Weishaar, 1989), anxiety (Salkovskis and Clarke, 1986) and schizophrenia (Frith, 1979) have all been conceptualized in this way, the assumption being that maladaptive thinking patterns, termed negative schemas, irrational thoughts, faulty cognitions or styles of attribution, are the cause of psychopathology. The cognitions are deemed to have a direct effect on the person's mood, on their view of the world, and the way they act within it. Thus Joan's, Deborah's or Simon's symptoms could be seen as being the result of faulty cognitions, negative and irrational thoughts and beliefs about themselves and about the world.

The cognitive approach looks to a number of key concepts in order to describe behaviour, including: information processing; beliefs and belief systems; memory, attitudes and expectations; self-statements; attributions; perception of helplessness and control; expectancy; mental representations; self-efficacy; problem solving; coping. These concepts are then used directly in therapy in order to ameliorate distress (Brewin, 1990).

Family therapy

These approaches all place emphasis on the individual as the focus of attention, a view which is challenged by the growth of family therapies, based on the premise that it is not *individuals* that are mad but the systems within which we live. Thus systems theory (Selvini-Palazzoli *et al.*, 1978), in which dysfunctions within a system are seen as being manifested by one person, the 'scapegoat', has become influential in health care. It is argued that the individual who is designated as mad is merely manifesting the problems which are present within the family, and thus treating her in isolation will not be of any help. It is the family which needs to be treated, with the therapist working at changing the troubled relationships so that the symptoms disappear. Within this framework, Simon's symptoms might be seen as resulting from difficulties within his family, as might Joan's depression.

Whilst psychoanalytic, cognitive-behavioural and family approaches are the dominant paradigms in operation in the mental health professions of today, other theories and therapies which might be adopted include humanistic therapy, group therapy, feminist therapy and a whole range of what a recent textbook deems 'innovative therapies' including primal integration therapy, encounter, co-counselling, psychodrama, bioenergetics, biosynthesis, psychosynthesis, transpersonal therapy, and neuro-linguistic programming (Rowan and Dryden, 1988).

SOCIOCULTURAL CRITIQUES

It might appear that the only controversy in the mental health field is that associated with the type of theory adopted, and the subsequent interventions offered for distress, but this is not the case. There have been many criticisms of the very notion of mental illness and the principles of labelling and diagnosis which underlie the classificatory system. It has been argued that what is deemed madness is a social construct, not an illness, and that to conceptualize distress as evidence of an underlying psychopathology is to scapegoat and blame the individual, whilst absolving society of responsibility. Different critics (Ussher, 1991, Chapter 6) have argued that the label of madness is merely a means of dismissing those who do not conform to current social rules, and thus 'what is peculiar in one situation may well be "normal" in another' (Barnes and Berke, 1971, p. 80). Evidence that definitions of psychopathology vary across cultures supports this view.

The mental health professions have been criticized for individualizing problems and oppressing those who do not fit in; acting as an agent of social control under the guise of care. As one critic argued, 'The role that psychology plays in legitimating the oppression of this society is by no means minor' (Brooks, 1973, p. 317). Evidence that more women, ethnic minorities and working class people are likely to receive a psychiatric diagnosis (Ussher, 1991) is used to support the view that psychopathology is merely a means of legitimizing the oppression of these individuals, and dismissing their resulting distress as internal illness.

Sociocultural critiques do not necessarily negate the suffering of individuals but biological or psychological processes are not seen as the root cause. Instead, social difficulties such as poor housing, lack of social support, economic factors and general social oppression are seen as leading to symptomatology. Social and political change is often then seen as the solution, not individual therapy. However, recent critics have incorporated these critiques into their clinical work, allowing both therapeutic intervention and acknowledgement of sociocultural realities. (See Ussher and Nicolson (1992) for a review in relation to gender issues.) These may involve professionals working with a wide range of factors in therapeutic intervention, including acknowledgement of social difficulties, economic reality, and often issues such as racism and sexism.

INTEGRATING THEORIES, THERAPIES AND CRITIQUES

A complex array of theories, therapies and critiques faces the individual professional attempting to provide answers to those in distress. Whilst there may seem to be little agreement and many conflicting opinions, a number of conclusions can safely be reached.

Firstly, there are significant numbers of individuals who at some time in their lives experience symptoms that cause distress to themselves or to their families. That distress is always framed and understood within the framework of the society in which it occurs, and in Western industrialized society today will be deemed psychopathology, madness or mental illness. This can be helpful for the individual if it results in access to care, empowering therapy or social change; it can be damaging if the individual is dismissed as 'ill', their opinions ignored (as is often the case with those diagnosed as 'mad'), and factors in their environment which might have led to distress disregarded.

The psychiatric classifications may be helpful in allowing comparison across individuals and in providing a meaningful label for those in distress, but they should not be reified and seen to exist as real entities in themselves. For example, depression does not cause an individual to feel suicidal, or to be unable to work. Depression is merely the label applied to a range of symptoms which might have a number of different causes. Equally, it is important to know that there is often disagreement between experts as to the appropriate diagnostic category in which to place an individual – a person diagnosed as depressed by one professional may be diagnosed as schizophrenic by another. So diagnosis and classification are not as clearcut as might first appear.

On the subject of aetiological explanation and therapeutic intervention, there are clearly many disagreements between professionals. What is essential is that an individual is informed of the various options open to them, and not merely offered one panacea (often pharmacological) which may not be appropriate. Equally, it is important to acknowledge the complex roots of distress, the social, psychological and biological concomitants of symptoms, and not to elevate one set of causal explanations above all others. Those who come forward for treatment from mental health professionals may benefit from change in a number of areas of their lives and, following consultation with the individual and often the family, this can be facilitated in an empowering way. The acknowledgement that intervention needs to take place within a multidisciplinary framework is one way of facilitating such change.

CONCLUSION

Many theories and therapies compete for prominence in the marketplace of the mad. In order to negotiate these different approaches, it is essential for the individual who experiences distress to have sufficient information in order to allow an informed choice between the range of therapeutic options currently available, or to be able to choose the option of no professional intervention at all.

REFERENCES

Barnes, M. and Berke, J. (1971) *Mary Barnes: Two Accounts of a Journey through Madness*, Macgibbon and Kee, London.

Baruch, G. and Treacher, A. (1978) *Psychiatry Observed*, Routledge and Kegan Paul, London.

Beck, A. and Weishaar, M. (1989) Cognitive therapy, in R. Corsini and D. Wedding (eds.) *Current Psychotherapies*, 4th edn, FE Peacock, Illinois.

Brewin, C. (1990) *Cognitive Foundations of Clinical Psychology*, 2nd edn, Lawrence Erlbaum, London.

Brooks, K. (1973) Freudianism is not a basis for Marxist psychology, in P. Brown (ed.) *Radical Psychology*, Tavistock, London.

Casement, P. (1985) *Learning from the Patient*, Tavistock, London.

Foucault, M. (1967) *Madness and Civilization: A history of insanity in the age of reason*, Tavistock, London.

Frith, C. (1979) Consciousness, information processing and schizophrenia, *British Journal of Psychiatry*, **134**, 225–35.

Gold, N. (1986) *The Good News about Depression*, Bantam Books, New York.

Malan, D.H. (1979) *Individual Psychotherapy and the Science of Psychodynamics*, Tavistock, Boston.

Porter, R. (1987) *Mind-Forg'd Manacles*, Athlone Press, London.

Rowan, J. and Dryden, W. (1988) *Innovative Therapy in Britain*, Open University Press, Milton Keynes.

Salkovskis, P. and Clarke, D. (1986) Cognitive and physiological approaches in the maintenance and treatment of panic attacks, in I. Hand and H. Wittchen (eds.) *Panic and Phobias*, Springer-Verlag, Berlin.

Scull, A.T. (1979) *Museums of Madness: The social organization of insanity in the nineteenth century*, Allen Lane, London.

Selvini-Palazzoli, M., Cecchin, G., Boscolo, L. and Prata, G. (1978) *Paradox and Counterparadox*, Jason Aronson, New York.

Ussher, J.M. (1991) *Women's Madness: Misogyny or mental illness?* Harvester Wheatsheaf, Hemel Hempstead.

Ussher, J.M. and Nicolson, P. (1992) *Gender Issues in Clinical Psychology*, Routledge, London.

12

Gender issues in ageing

Paula Nicolson

INTRODUCTION

Ageing is an increasingly important issue for counsellors and health professionals, not only because as a population we are living longer than 20 years ago, but because middle-aged adults expect much more of their lives. While both longer life and increased expectations are positive, paradoxically they precipitate practical problems for the health services and emotional and social problems for individuals and their families.

In this chapter I focus upon the ways in which increased capacities and expectations from mid-life onwards create potential 'crises', and specifically explore the different issues faced by women and men. I begin by reviewing psychological knowledge on gender and mid to late adulthood, including both the social and intellectual aspects of growing older. A critique of the 'ageing equals deterioration' model in psychology is offered and the distinction between female and male life courses and potential milestones is made explicit. The psychological knowledge which traditionally informs professional practice is based upon an apparently gender-free and (by default) male model of growing older. In this chapter the gender issues in ageing are made clear, specifically in the context of understanding professional practice with older clients.

GENDER

Sex and gender impinge upon our lives even before conception. Almost all parents have fantasies and expectations about the sex of their child and following safe delivery, their main concern is with the infant's sex (Leonard, 1984). This 'labelling' marks the beginning of the development of gender identity, which distinguishes the life cycles of women and men in a number of ways. Unfortunately most psychological studies of the life cycle, middle age and ageing have concentrated on men's lives (Erikson, 1950; Levinson, 1986); it is only recently that psychology has considered gender to be important and identified women's lives as having an independent validity, rather than as just 'different' from men's (Nicolson and Ussher, 1992).

Although there are different patterns of behaviour and expectations for girls and boys and women and men from infancy, it is only the first 30 years of life which have been well documented (mainly because of differential reproductive roles and family relationships: see Chapter 6). From mid-life onwards, most studies fail to distinguish women's experience from men's, other than in relation to biology (i.e. the menopause) and reproductive arrangements (i.e. children leaving home).

LATER LIFE

Erik Erikson's model of the 'Eight Ages of Man' identified a series of stages of psychological and social development through the life cycle which coincided with biological age. Each psychological stage of development took place alongside a social task (for example, leaving school) or a biological one (for example, puberty) and in any society there is a 'cog-wheeling' of life cycles. This means that when individuals want to become parents, nurture and provide for others, this desire meshes with their infants' and pre-school children's needs at their own particular developmental stage.

Erikson perceived developmental change to be accompanied by 'crises'. Following adolescence, where individuals establish a sense of identity, and young adulthood, when they become able to form intimate relationships with others, middle and late adulthood have their own distinct tasks and crises. He called these two stages 'generativity versus stagnation/self-absorption' (mid-life), and 'integrity versus despair and disgust' (old age).

For Erikson the mid-life stage was about finding a means of contributing to future generations – via work or having a family. Old age was about coming to terms with impending death and re-evaluating the life that led up to that point. Despair in old age coincided with a self-appraisal of missed opportunity, waste, guilt and lack of integrity.

Despite introducing the notion of the whole life (rather than taking from Freud and Piaget the emphasis on childhood as the only period of psychological consequence), Erikson still only identified two stages of development from mid-life on. Also, despite acknowledging cultural and gender differences, he *dismisses* girls and women as having different experience from the 'normal' at each stage, so that, apart from parenting, women are invisible in Erikson's schema. However, Erikson must be acknowledged for placing the notions of mid-life and old age upon the psychological agenda as periods of interest, not just part of a process of deterioration.

Mid-life

Levinson's (1978, 1986) work was influential in bringing the notion of the *mid-life crisis* to the fore and legitimating a number of apparently 'out of character' behaviours and anxieties that had implications for individuals' psychological and physiological health. According to Levinson, mid-life transitions begin around the age of 40, and in his research 80% of the respondents experienced emotional struggles and upheavals within themselves and in their social and work relationships. They were angry, resentful, felt themselves to be irrational, anxious and guilty and often made dramatic changes in order to cope with this. For example, they left their jobs, had an affair, changed their style of dress, took up hobbies which forced them to have new kinds of experiences with different people and so on (see Chapter 3).

Levinson's respondents were all men and subsequent studies of this period of mid-life crisis similarly were mainly about men. Studies of women in mid-life and old age traditionally focus upon the biological changes brought about by the menopause. The assumptions here have been that, at this time, women lose their social and sexual value. Such a view, however, has been firmly challenged by feminist psychologists (for example, Hunter, 1990). Women have also been portrayed as experiencing the 'empty nest' syndrome, being left by grown-up children and even by their partners. Whereas mid-life for men is a crisis, mid-life for women is seen as 'terminal' or at least the beginning of the end! But does such an image stand up to evidence? If not, where does the image come from?

Certainly most evidence would suggest that women who are elderly now (in the 1990s) live longer than their male contemporaries and adjust better to old age than do men. Is this because their lives after the age of around 40 are somehow even and unstressful or is it because systematic studies of women's lives had previously been neglected, forcing us to rely on stereotypes? These questions need serious consideration by individuals in the helping professions in order to provide appropriate care.

Old age

Old age is potentially a time of regret and physical ill health, dependence, loneliness and poverty, and indeed counsellors and health care workers are most likely to see the people for whom this is the case. The persistent image of old age is indeed so negative that many care workers prefer to work with other age groups. Stereotypes of the elderly also suggest a broad pattern of intellectual deterioration, loss of memory, hearing, sight and mobility impairment and, sadly, many old people are treated as having multiple social and psychological deficiencies. While there is some truth in all of this and some people, particularly women, are subject to Alzheimer's disease, it is also true that psychologists have begun slowly to realize a number of ways in which our stereotypes of the elderly have developed from poorly structured research or insufficient evidence.

Rabbit's (1988) work on thinking in old age suggests that although memory deteriorates with age, there is little apparent difference in performance between people in their 50s and 60s and those in their late 70s. With a sensible awareness on the part of older individuals that they need to take account of *some* memory loss and adopt 'aides memoires', most can combat this deterioration. Rabbit also suggests that part of the distress suffered by the elderly is caused by their own self-image. Thus ageism itself can have negative effects. If negative images of the elderly are the only ones available and everyone treats old people as generally deficient, this in itself will precipitate psychological distress, possibly leading to further social and emotional problems. But where do 'ageist' ideas come from?

Kimmel (1990) suggested that previous psychological research, generalized from cross-sectional studies, produced a broad picture of universal deterioration in intellect, memory, and cognitive skills after mid-life. Individual subjects in such research potentially varied in abilities from the very competent to the much less so. Taking the average ability as the main measure appeared to bring about a picture of decline for the whole sample.

This kind of research evidence has passed into popular Western mythology giving rise to images of ageing and deterioration, in contrast to many Eastern cultures who value the wisdom of older people. Through longitudinal studies, individuals' differences in competence clearly emerge so that someone competent in their youth and middle age would probably remain so. Like every other 'muscle', exercising intellectual faculties ensures their endurance!

GENDER THROUGHOUT THE LIFECYCLE

While we must acknowledge important psychological changes from mid-life onwards, it may be more realistic to see them as development rather than deterioration. Psychological studies have previously been guilty of influencing our attitudes in this way so that all change post-adolescence is seen as regression, decline or deterioration (Salmon, 1985).

The older we become, the more experience of life and self-knowledge we possess. It may be that we have endured crises or perhaps have experienced undue distress through life events and feel less happy than in our younger years. Health care workers and counsellors can help individuals with adjustment in these areas and provide positive insights. In this chapter I acknowledge the differential psychological implications of gender, and although these have both biological and social origins, I argue that it is social expectations that frame biological experience. The differential value placed on particular achievements (for example parenthood, employment and promotion) appear to be weighted according to gender, and health professionals need to be aware that these are social constructions rather than 'intrinsic' qualities.

Men and the life cycle

By mid-life men are expected to be married, fathers, and at the height of a successful career. Because many men do not conform to this model, they experience distress, as do many men who have behaved in the prescribed ways only to experience them as stressful. For example, a man may be married but it might not be a successful partnership, he might be gay and considered a deviant, he might not be able to have or want to have children, he might be divorced, unemployed, disabled and have no chance of a career – successful or otherwise. However, this archetypal norm persists and men, for want of an alternative, measure themselves against this.

Men and employment

Because of the social pressures on men as breadwinners, the issue of paid employment is most salient for men in mid-life and in old age. Prior to the age of 40 it is possible to change or lose a job without fear of exclusion from employment or even a career, but physical labour is more difficult for many after mid-life. This often means taking work which is less well paid or not finding work at all. How often have white collar employees been faced with job application information which excludes the over-35s? There is a clear assumption on the part of employers that from 38 to 40 men's stamina, strength, professional growth, intellectual agility and flexibility have diminished. As suggested above, however, this is not based upon a systematic review of psychological evidence but myth, and although there is now legislation in the USA and EC countries to combat such practices, this has not so far been effective in the United Kingdom. The prejudice of employers against older workers gives some individuals a sense of failure (Nicolson and Phillips, 1990; Phillips and Nicolson, 1990).

Men and sexuality

Until relatively recently psychological research on sexuality concentrated on adolescence and young adulthood. The implication is that once an individual developed the capacity for sex, within an intimate relationship, this became an area of life in which they felt confident and capable. The increase in the divorce rate and mid-life loneliness have clarified a number of doubts and troubles facing mid-life and elderly men which are qualitatively different from earlier experiences. It is tempting to 'dispose' of changes in desire and arousal patterns as part of biological ageing, but ageing accounts for only a small propor-tion of changes in men's sexuality in mid-life and beyond. Most psychological research emphasizes the centrality of sexual in-tercourse in men's sexual lives. Scientific data about patterns of arousal, orgasm and resolution (Masters and Johnson, 1966) seem to be the popular determinant of virility. The relationship aspect of sexuality is frequently neglected in explaining men's sexual problems and anxieties, and men's need for affection, warmth and companionship are often ignored. It is important for health professionals to realize the intrinsic link between sex, warmth and affection. Often because of social pressures, men might express loneliness and need for comfort as the need for sex. It is important that men are not just seen as needing to fulfil a 'biological drive' but that they themselves, for reasons of socialization, may find their more emotional needs harder to express.

Studies of sexual intercourse during the course of a relation-ship (usually a marriage, once again the norm for men in mid-life, specifically the once-married heterosexual father) sug-gest that the average man reports a decline in the frequency of intercourse in his 50s and 60s (see Pfeiffer and Davis, 1974) and this is often attributed to a reduced biological capacity. This needs to be questioned because when a decline in sexual activ-ity is perceived as a 'problem' or an aspect of the ageing process, it often leads to unnecessary emotional stress.

As with intellectual decline, there is a range of individual differences in enjoyment and interest in sexual intercourse, so that some men willingly stop or reduce their sexual activities while others do not. Any counsellor or health professional working with a man with this self-identified problem needs to establish the individual's own interest and capacity rather than assess their client in terms of an age-related norm. It is also important to disentangle the individual's idea of what he thinks he should be doing from what he himself really wants! Most recent psychological research suggests that sex is of positive benefit for men if they want to engage in it and have a reciprocal relationship with an enthusiastic partner, but there are no universal guidelines for what constitutes 'normal' behaviour.

Reduced sexual desire is more likely to be a consequence of a poor relationship or depression for other reasons than a symptom of ageing. Divorce and the break-up of any sexual partnership is problematic, not only sexually but socially and emotionally, and may lead a man to consider himself undesirable or unattractive, which further reduces self-esteem.

WOMEN AND THE LIFECYCLE

Women's invisibility in all spheres of psychological life has meant that knowledge of women's experiences of ageing has been limited to being a counterpart to male ageing. This is further compounded by the preponderance of male psychologists with their male-centred ideas who describe women's lives both in relation to men and as men think they should be (see Nicolson and Ussher, 1992). The yardstick of 'normal' development has been based upon men's ideas.

That is, women's assumed traditional life patterns of work, marriage, motherhood, part-time work and retirement when her male partner retires is not what happens to most women. Women may be lesbian or choose not to marry or to have children, may be infertile, become single parents, get divorced at any stage or have a career and be a working mother and wife. There are several other permutations too!

Women in the family

At mid-life, women do tend to focus on their reproductive capacity, particularly if they are childless, because there is a biological limit to their reproductive life. However, because of greater personal control over fertility, women at mid-life may be at any one of a range of stages in relation to their childbearing. They may have children about to leave home. They may be starting a second family with a new partner. They may be having a baby for the first time and increasingly, they may be separating or divorcing from a partner (see Chapter 7).

Mid-life also coincides with parental ageing and because of women's traditional role in the family as mother, without a full-time career or 'serious' job, they tend to take over the care of elderly relatives – both their own and/or their partners'. Finch and Groves (1983) address the ways in which caring for others circumscribes women's lives.

While this pattern of caring is true for many from early adulthood, particularly if they become mothers then, it is exacerbated from mid-life onwards. Just as women begin to see the chance to spend time, thought and other resources on themselves, with the growing independence of their children, their caring capacities are charged to the full once again. This can extend to caring for elderly neighbours as well as relatives.

Health professionals are often involved, particularly through community care programmes, in ensuring that women remain in this role. Women are pressured, albeit in a subtle way, to maintain their caring status. How often, when the care of an elderly person is being discussed, is the question asked 'Does she have any relatives?'. This almost inevitably means 'female' relatives as the male is generally perceived as unable to care because of his working role.

Some women are also tied to their partner's working role, particularly if that (male) partner is in business, the armed services, a politician or a clergyman (Finch, 1983). Some men's work actually has a direct requirement for a wife. Unmarried Prime Ministers, for example Edward Heath, are not popular and the wife of a President in the USA has a very distinct role. For most women, though, the role of clergyman's wife or businessman's wife, with the overt demands on their time and talents, is binding but paradoxically invisible. Divorce under these conditions at mid-life not only disrupts the family but deprives the woman of a 'career'.

Women and employment

Recent demographic changes have provoked government-backed employers' initiatives to encourage women into the workforce, particularly women at mid-life with experience and training prior to becoming mothers. Women's employment patterns traditionally differ from men's although when it comes to promotion and reaching the top in any area, employment breaks often militate against success. Because of women's broadly based caring responsibilities, with which they often cope alongside their jobs, it may be that female identities are not so bound up with a particular job as perhaps is the case with men. This cannot be taken for granted, though.

Between 1970 and 1980 women entered previously male-dominated work of all kinds (for example, management, farming, construction and sales) and it is likely that their commitment to this work is equal to that of men (Kimmel, 1990). There is some evidence that this has been accompanied by an increased commitment of the male partner to childcare and domestic tasks (Lewis, 1986) but this is not always clearcut (Nicolson, 1990).

There is now some public awareness that women's entry into a career may be later than that of men, but that they can still be successful (Nicolson and Phillips, 1991). The life cycle point of crisis for men at mid-life, when they re-evaluate their contribution and potential for success at work, coincides with the stage at which women may be enthusiastically entering a career with a vision of a future.

It is a fallacy to suggest that the age of 40 marks a decline in career growth. That may be the case with men. It is only recently that some equal opportunities legislation has been introduced to help women. In the UK it is still difficult to enter an academic job over the age of 30, with the assumption of a first degree and PhD prior to that (Nicolson and Phillips, 1991).

Retirement problems for women have traditionally been limited to having to cope with a male partner's presence in the home. This is no longer always the case and women are likely to experience a similar sense of loss and anxiety on retirement as men. However, in terms of re-evaluation of their lives, women who have worked and have caring involvements may be less likely to experience 'despair' than 'integrity'.

Women and sexuality

Women's sexual performance has never been perceived as declining with mid-life in the way that men's has. However, it is women's attractiveness that has been a major issue and has been seen as so important that women will go to great lengths to attempt to sustain what they perceive as physical desirability, such as plastic surgery, extremes of diet and more recently the contentious hormone replacement therapy (HRT). But why should women be perceived as less attractive as they grow older? Itzin (1986) and Ferguson (1983) have shown how media images of women and femininity stress a very specific notion of what constitutes sexual attractiveness. It is also a standard joke that only women well under 30 are desirable.

The emphasis in popular (and even serious) newspapers and TV programmes on women's appearance and how to stay young serves to reinforce this and persuades women to internalize their own sense of being 'past it' at 40. For some, the feeling of distance from the sexual arena provides the chance to 'relax' about their sexuality, but it leaves many feeling hopeless and desperate, particularly if they have lived with a male partner who has left them for the proverbial younger woman.

The coincidence in timing of the menopause and the 'empty nest' leaves women feeling literally on the sexual scrap heap and may have the effect of making them neglect themselves in every way; not simply in terms of staying slim or not keeping up a good hairstyle but neglecting to look after their physical and mental health, which leads to further depression and reduced self-confidence. Health care workers and counsellors may have been alerted to women's vulnerability at mid-life but need to identify with women clients a range of ways in which self-confidence may be restored. This in itself can lead to renewed sexual and emotional energy. Even without the aid of HRT, the notion of the menopause as negative and marking the end of sexual activity is a spurious myth. Women themselves at this time often identify as 'asexual' but this again is more a result of the media and other public images than hormones.

Many health practitioners see HRT as a panacea for depression and unrequited sexual desire or lack of sexual attractiveness in women of mid-life to old age (Hunter, 1990). However, it is more important to enable women to see the potential in their lives as people – workers, carers, partners and sexual beings – than to label them as cases for treatment, which is the effect of proposing HRT.

LOSS IN MID-LIFE AND OLD AGE

Any developmental changes may be perceived as loss in that adolescence is a lost innocence and young adulthood equates with the loss of dependency and being cared for by parents. However, losses such as these through the life cycle give access to potential psychological gains as well. Marris (1986), in his book *Loss and Change*, argued theoretically and intuitively that losses potentially lead to psychological growth and reintegration. Thus loss precedes and is part of psychological development. While this remains true, sometimes loss in mid-life and old age may be unrelenting and fundamental. The gradual loss of capabilities may well be perceived by some individuals as a great problem, but the loss of life partner, parents, friends, children, a working life, income, health or mobility may become imminent at mid-life. As old age approaches, the more often individuals may be faced with death and the more they are likely to become aware of the reality of their own death and possibly repress or deny this.

Death of a partner

While there are a number of potential losses which have their greatest impact in mid-life and old age (mentioned above), I concentrate here particularly upon the death of a partner, although clearly there are psychological parallels with the effects of divorce (see Chapter 7). Early interest in the psychology of bereavement focused upon widows (for example, Murray Parkes, 1980), at least in part because widowhood is more common than widowerhood. For example, in the USA in 1984, 366,000 men between 55 and 64 were widowed compared with 2,054,000 women. Men die younger and the USA Bureau of Census in 1986 estimated that widowhood is six times more likely for women in mid-life (i.e. 35 to 54) than for men.

Marris's early study of widows (1958) demonstrated that loneliness, social isolation and reduced income were problems faced by widows in addition to the actual grief for their lost partner. The younger the widow, the more likely it is that she will have dependent children, which intensifies certain practical problems while potentially alleviating some emotional aspects of the process. Murray Parkes' (1980) study of the bereavement process in widows was useful in developing a model to understand normal grieving, and vital for counsellors and health workers as it demonstrated the length, depth and variability of the normal grieving cycle (see Nicolson and Bayne, 1990, for a discussion of this).

Although specific studies of gender differences in grieving are inconclusive (Demi, 1989), knowledge of women's and men's life cycles enables us to make certain predictions about differences. For widows it is clearly often the case that much of their income, identity and status has been derived from their male partners and thus losing that partner is a multi-deprivation. Men who lose a female partner are not so likely to suffer the same kind of loss. However, recent psychological feminist literature would suggest that women experience subordination of their status and individuality in marriage, so that the death of a spouse may potentially lead to independence, perhaps for the first time for some women. This identifies potential for psychological growth, and indeed Murray Parkes' evidence would support this. Even widowhood in old age is not the end of psychological and emotional development. Human individuals may be capable of greater scope in behaviour and emotion than most put into practice.

For men, losing their partner often means losing their emotional, social and practical supports. Men in the current cohort of the elderly, for example, are unlikely to have any practical domestic skills, such as housekeeping, shopping or cooking. Their immediate emotional needs will also be neglected unless an adult daughter or other female relative is available. Social needs may be met at a club or pub but this varies according to social class, and many men would have gained contact at work or through their wives' arrangements.

Health care workers often find themselves supplying domestic and practical support to men without any physical reason. Because of the low social status attributed to domestic activities, men are often resistant to them and look for a woman's help (home help, housekeeper, cleaning lady or new partner) in order to survive. This presents a dilemma for health care workers for which individuals need to seek their own, often compromising solutions.

Middle-aged widowers, as with divorcees, seek remarriage as quickly as possible while their female contemporaries often value their freedom from domestic drudgery and avoid remarriage, attempting to establish alternative social networks or new patterns with a different partner (Bernard, 1974).

Lesbians and gay men are often overlooked in terms of understanding the loss of a partner and it is hopefully unnecessary to say how similar problems and distresses are equally true for them and indeed may be exacerbated by outmoded social prejudices which fail to give them 'permission' to mourn.

COUNSELLING IN MID-LIFE

Understanding the differential impact of the mid-life crisis on women and men is vital. Individuals themselves have different kinds of concerns, but for men the life course pattern suggests that mid-life is a time to re-evaluate work and sexuality (Levinson, 1986). For women, attitudes and experience of work and family life are more variable and their anxieties, regrets and distress have a potentially broader base. Although the concept of a mid-life crisis, or transitional stage, is useful, it should not be employed to label a problem. Different people need to be helped to operate different coping strategies in order to come to terms with all the variations of their first 40 or so years.

Gender divisions are deeply embedded in almost all cultures and thus difficult to challenge. What is important is that individuals are supported when they themselves challenge the norms. For example, older women wanting to work or have active sexual relationships may well consider themselves 'deviant' and therefore need support in their chosen behaviour. Similarly men who are unemployed at mid-life can choose to focus on domestic tasks, but need support for this choice, rather than to be forced to adjust to social requirements. It is very easy for all of us, however aware of gender issues we consider ourselves to be, to fall into stereotypical beliefs in relation to the middle-aged to elderly. This is tied in with ideas that older people are set in their ways and cannot change and that they represent and support the status quo. This is no more likely to be true of older people than it is of younger generations. Health professionals, as far as possible, need to challenge their *own* assumptions about older people and their capacities and experiences in mid-life and beyond.

CONCLUSIONS

Psychologists have only recently begun to re-evaluate their ideas about adulthood, ageing and deterioration. Rather than asking how soon does psychological deterioration occur, researchers now focus on effectiveness. If some psychological capacities, such as short term memory, are vulnerable to ageing, then how may they be protected and supported?

Individuals encouraged to develop throughout life are less likely to experience psychological deterioration than others who are not. We are, however, all vulnerable to the myths about growing older. Health professionals often contribute to these by referring to older clients and patients as 'old dears' or 'little old ladies' and so on. Mid-life and old age are periods of intense change and potentially periods of growth rather than decay, provided there are adequate social and emotional supports and if ageism can be challenged successfully.

Assumptions that a normal life cycle is a male life cycle have now been challenged. Feminists within psychology have argued that women's life cycles should be seen as different from men's, rather than 'deviant'. In many ways women have greater potential for a variety of experience and psychological growth than do men because they are not so bound by the social constraints imposed by 'masculinity' (Archer, 1989).

Any understanding of human ageing, then, has to account for biology, psychology and social factors and these need to be contextualized within a framework that takes account of gender. Professional intervention is more likely to be effective if it takes all these factors into account, as well as the growing awareness that there is life after 40!

REFERENCES

Archer, J. (1989) Childhood gender roles: structure and development, *The Psychologist*, **9**, 367–70.
Bernard, J. (1974) *The Future of Marriage*, Pelican, Harmondsworth.
Demi, A.S. (1989) Death of a spouse, In R.A. Kalish (ed.) *Midlife Loss: Coping strategies*, Sage, London.
Erikson, E. (1950) *Childhood and Society*, Norton, New York.
Ferguson, M. (1983) *Forever Feminine: Women's magazines and the cult of femininity*, Heinemann, London.
Finch, J. (1983) *Married to the Job*, George Allen and Unwin, London.
Finch, J. and Groves, D. (1983) *A Labour of Love: Women, work and caring*, Routledge and Kegan Paul, London.
Hunter, M. (1990) Sexuality and the menopause, paper presented at the BPS London Conference, City University, as part of the Psychology and Biology of Female Sexual Behaviour Symposium.
Itzin, C. (1986) Media images of women: the social construction of

ageism and sexism, In S. Wilkinson (ed.) *Feminist Social Psychology: Developing theory and practice,* Open University Press, Milton Keynes.

Kimmel, D.C. (1990) *Adulthood and Ageing: An interdisciplinary developmental view,* Wiley, New York.

Leonard, P. (1984) *Personality and Ideology,* Macmillan, Basingstoke.

Levinson, D. (1978) *The Seasons of a Man's Life,* Knopf, New York.

Levinson, D. (1986) The conception of adult development, *American Psychologist,* **41**, 3–13.

Lewis, C. (1986) *Becoming a Father,* Open University Press, Milton Keynes.

Marris, P. (1958) *Widows and their Families,* Routledge and Kegan Paul, London.

Marris, P. (1986) *Loss and Change,* Routledge and Kegan Paul, London.

Masters, W.H. and Johnson, V.E. (1966) *Human Sexual Response,* J. and A. Churchill Ltd, London.

Murray Parkes, C. (1980) *Bereavement,* Pelican, Harmondsworth.

Nicolson, P. (1990) A brief report of women's expectations of men's behaviour in the transition to parenthood: contradictions and conflicts for counselling psychology practice, *Counselling Psychology Quarterly,* **3**, no.4, 353–62.

Nicolson, P. and Bayne, R. (1990) *Applied Psychology for Social Workers,* 2nd edn, Macmillan, London.

Nicolson, P. and Phillips, E.M. (1990) Ageism and academia, *The Psychologist,* **3**, no.9, 393–5.

Nicolson, P. and Ussher, J.M. (1992) *The Psychology of Women's Health and Health Care,* Macmillan, London.

Pfeiffer, E. and Davis, G.C. (1974) Determinants of sexual behaviour in middle and old age, in E. Palmore (ed.) *Normal Ageing,* Duke University Press, Durham, D.C.

Phillips, E.M. and Nicolson, P. (1990) Declining intelligence or applied wisdom, paper presented at the BPS London Conference, City University.

Rabbit, P. (1988) Social psychology, neurosciences and cognitive psychology need each other (and gerontology needs all three of them), *The Psychologist,* **1**, 500–506.

Salmon, P. (1985) *Living in Time,* J.M. Dent and Sons, London.

13

AIDS and psychology

Keith Phillips

INTRODUCTION

A decade has passed since initial reports appeared of the first few cases of young men suffering a rare form of pneumonia indicative of damage to their immune systems. This was the first evidence that Acquired Immune Deficiency Syndrome (AIDS) had arrived. It has since become pandemic.

Psychology has a major role to play in the fight against AIDS. Interventions to prevent the further spread of AIDS will involve social workers, health practitioners and other professional groups. Counsellors will be called upon to assist the management of the disease for patients and their carers. This chapter will explore just some of the ways in which these professionals increasingly will come into contact with the personal tragedies of the AIDS epidemic. But first some brief background.

The World Health Organization to date has recorded 345,000 cases of AIDS worldwide from more than 160 different countries. It estimates that when under-reporting by some countries and underdiagnosis by others are taken into account, there may already have been more than one million cases of AIDS. By the year 2000 it is predicted there will be 30–40 million individuals infected with the Human Immunodeficiency Virus (HIV). It is this virus that is responsible for weakening the body's immune defences, making it vulnerable to the opportunistic illnesses that characterize AIDS – pneumonias and cancers. The situation in the UK is serious too. Since reporting began in 1982 the number of AIDS cases has increased steadily to the June 1991 level of 4758. It is estimated that there are at least three times this number of individuals infected with HIV in the UK. Many of these will develop AIDS within a few years.

TRANSMISSION OF HIV

HIV has been identified in many different body fluids including blood, sexual fluids, saliva, tears and breast milk. However, the virus is only poorly transmitted and there is no evidence that infection can occur by purely social contacts such as working in the same environment or sharing cutlery and utensils. There are only three effective routes for transmission of the virus from one individual to another. They are: by transfer of infected blood (e.g. during transfusions, or by the unsterilized needles or syringes used to inject drugs) or of blood products (as occurred with UK haemophiliacs given untreated clotting factor VIII); via sexual fluids during unprotected penetrative sexual intercourse, or by transfer from mother to foetus pre-natally or post-natally during breast feeding. The probability of transmission by these routes (or level of risk) varies considerably. In some instances the risk can be eliminated entirely; for example, by screening blood and blood products there can be total elimination of transmission via medical procedures. Behavioural transmission through sexual intercourse or injecting drugs is more difficult to deal with.

Historically the first cases of AIDS in the West were diagnosed among male homosexuals and later injecting drug users too. Representations of AIDS in the media helped establish the myth that AIDS was confined to minority groups that were stigmatized as being deviant or marginalized in other ways. The myth persists despite what is known about the transmission of HIV and the epidemiological evidence from Africa where AIDS is a heterosexual disease affecting as many women as men. Worldwide, it is estimated that 70% of all HIV infections are the result of sexual transmission between men and women. There are no 'groups' at risk for AIDS, there are only individuals who engage in risk-associated behaviours. For example, for sexual transmission, anal intercourse is associated with higher risk of HIV infection than vaginal intercourse though in both instances use of a condom will reduce the risk considerably (though not eliminate it entirely).

AIDS is an issue for anyone engaging in sexual intercourse or injecting drugs, women and men alike. Indeed, in the UK the rate of increase of HIV infection is now faster among women than men. Trends in the statistics are now beginning to confirm the message that health professionals have been pressing for some time – AIDS does not discriminate, it is a health issue for all. It must also be faced that as more women become infected with HIV, the instances of paediatric AIDS will increase, presenting additional problems for the health professions. The most recent statistics show that in London in 1991, there were three times as many infants born with HIV infection as in the previous year. The Medical Research Council's programme of anonymous testing of women attending antenatal clinics in Inner London found that one in 500 has antibodies to HIV. The impact of these statistics will become apparent during the next decade.

THE PRIMARY PREVENTION OF AIDS

Primary prevention of AIDS means preventing individuals from becoming infected with HIV by the elimination of those behaviours that allow transmission of the virus from one individual to another (Phillips, 1991). Behaviour modification, however, is not easily achieved which should not surprise us as the reasons why people change or fail to change their behaviours are complex and poorly understood. Models of behaviour change in health contexts are largely based upon the idea of a person as a rational decision-maker weighing the costs and benefits of engaging in a particular behaviour. These models have been only moderately successful in explaining health-related behaviour change. Despite this, the antecedents of behaviour emphasized by these models – information, attitudes, social norms, intentions – have received considerable investigation in relation to AIDS.

An early reaction to AIDS in the UK was the introduction of mass public education campaigns to inform people about AIDS. The campaigns have been conducted through television, radio and newspapers as well as leaflets to individual households. These campaigns and similar ones in other countries were extremely effective in raising awareness about the existence of AIDS. Unfortunately simply providing information has not proved to be effective in changing people's attitudes to the disease and has conspicuously failed to alter behaviour. Moreover, in many ways the presentation of information about AIDS by the media has helped confirm the myth that AIDS is confined to individuals who can be labelled as belonging to a deviant 'group', e.g. injecting drug users or male homosexuals, and therefore is not an issue for the general heterosexual population.

Mass campaigns therefore have only limited value. More specific programmes for behaviour change are required and there is evidence that these may be more successful. Interventions to prevent AIDS have focused attention upon those behaviours that allow transfer of bodily fluids which has resulted in programmes for injecting drug users (IDUs) and advice upon the adoption of safer sex.

AIDS is variously identified as a medical, public health, social, moral and economic issue. Programmes to limit the spread of AIDS must be sensitive to these different dimensions if they are to have any chance of producing significant changes in behaviour. There is increasing evidence that community-based interventions may be most effective though more evaluations of such programmes are urgently needed. Health professionals and social workers are ideally placed to play a role in community interventions. They must be supported by a comprehensive policy and the infrastructure to provide adequate resources (Coates, 1990). Interventions must provide communities not only with information but also the skill to encourage appropriate behaviour change for risk reduction together with a supportive and appropriate culture to facilitate and sustain change.

Two aspects that are important are the education of young people who are about to become sexually active and counselling adolescents and adults who are already sexually active about risk reduction.

Educating adolescents about AIDS

Adolescents are an important group for future AIDS education campaigns. They will inevitably wish to experience relationships of different kinds, non-intimate as well as intimate, and for many, their relationships will involve sexual activities. Some will experiment with drugs and of these a minority will inject drugs such as heroin or benzodiazepines. Adolescents need to acquire the skills to manage their sexual and drug-using behaviours. Information alone is not sufficient; they need to acquire social skills – negotiation, assertiveness, the language and skills to manage their sexual lives (White *et al.*, 1989) – and to develop the self-esteem necessary to take responsibility for their own health (see Chapter 3). A health education curriculum that includes sexual behaviours, contraception and AIDS could also make a significant contribution to moulding the beliefs and intentions of young people, enabling appropriate precautions against AIDS to be adopted. To achieve this early in their sexual or drug-using lives would be a significant step towards limiting the spread of AIDS among the next generation of young adults (Melton, 1988).

Risk reduction strategies

For adolescents and adults who are already engaging in sexual activities or are injecting drugs, the major objective of strategies against AIDS is to reduce the risk to themselves and their partners of HIV infection. To achieve risk reduction means persuading people to modify their behaviours. The particular behaviours to be changed vary from one individual to another which is why intervention programmes must be clearly targeted. Two aspects that have received particular attention are the harm minimization approach to injecting drug users (IDUs) accompanied by the introduction of syringe exchange schemes, and promotion of safer sex among both homosexual and heterosexual communities.

Injecting drug use

Of the 619 new cases of AIDS recorded in 1989/90 in the UK, 26% were attributable to injecting drug use. This reflects the consequence of risk behaviours that did exist among some IDUs. Sharing drug injecting equipment that is contaminated with blood infected with HIV is an effective way of transmitting the virus. Avoidance of sharing or adoption of safer practices such as sterilization of the equipment can eliminate transmission by this route. The indications are that the health promotion campaigns targeted at IDUs have been successful in this regard. There is increasing evidence that these messages to adopt harm minimization by avoiding sharing injecting equipment have been heeded and adopted by them (Mulleady *et al.*, 1990). The messages have been reinforced by practical policies that assist risk reduction, including the introduction of syringe exchange schemes and pharmacy exchanges where IDUs can return used injecting equipment and obtain sterile equipment free of charge. This public health approach not only assists risk reduction, it also brings the IDUs into contact with drug advice agencies and gives them the opportunity for more general health care. In addition, schemes in the USA based upon outreach programmes, where health workers locate IDUs in their own communities to offer health education and advice upon risk reduction, have also been effective in reducing the spread of HIV infection (Watters, 1989).

The exclusive emphasis upon this aspect of the IDUs' lives, however, may have been misplaced. If the IDU is sexually active then injecting drugs is not the only risk of transmission of HIV. The IDU may contract HIV from a sexual partner or may transmit to a partner. Some IDUs are at particular risk in this regard if they engage in prostitution in order to finance the purchase of drugs. The counselling offered to IDUs should not solely be concerned with their drug use; they need sexual counselling too. This presents a challenge to the counsellor and client alike and it may be that drugs counsellors need additional training in this regard (Mulleady *et al.*, 1990). There is evidence, however, that interventions based upon skills-building group sessions can be effective for reducing risk-related sexual behaviours among drug users (Schilling *et al.*, 1991).

Promoting safer sex

IDUs are not unique in requiring advice upon safer sex. AIDS is a public health issue for us all. The risks of HIV infection from sexual activities have been well publicized yet much remains to be done in this area. Sexual transmission is the most common route of transmission of HIV and health education about AIDS rightly reflects this. It is vital that safer sex be widely publicized if people are to be persuaded to adopt practices to minimize risk. Safer sex means eliminating the transfer of bodily fluids from one to another. This can be achieved in many ways including celibacy, non-penetrative sex, use of condoms during penetrative sex and avoiding practices that may damage tissues and cause transfer of blood.

Some people have changed their behaviours already. There is evidence that in the USA and UK, male homosexuals have achieved great changes towards risk reduction. Self-reports of behaviour change are confirmed by a reduction in sexually transmitted diseases and reduced rates of HIV infection amongst this group. The successful changes include reducing the number of sexual partners and avoidance of high risk activities. This does not mean, however, that the changes will be invariably maintained. A continuing programme of health promotion will be required to sustain the progress already made. It should also be recognized that counselling for risk reduction for those at risk or those infected with the virus will remain an important element of the primary prevention of AIDS.

COUNSELLING AND THE MANAGEMENT OF AIDS

Counselling is not only important for primary prevention. It became accepted as a central component of the management of AIDS from the earliest days of the pandemic (Green, 1989). There are many reasons why this is so. First, the emergence of AIDS coincided with an explosion of counselling practice and increasing acceptance of counselling as a treatment for a variety of disorders. Linked with this is the fact that it is probably easier to encourage a novel treatment when confronted with a novel disease. Thus counselling has become more acceptable for patients with AIDS than for some others with similarly life-threatening diseases such as cancer. Counselling may also play a role in maintaining good health for those infected with HIV. Most importantly perhaps, it seems that those with HIV want counselling and actively seek the support it provides. This is understandable given the reactions to AIDS in many societies where the infected individuals are stigmatized and marginalized. It should also be acknowledged that medical treatment of AIDS (e.g. with AZT or through hospitalization) is extremely expensive and, given the predicted increases in AIDS cases expected worldwide, counselling offers a response to the disease at relatively modest cost. In the developing countries counselling may be both effective and perhaps the only realistic option if medical resources are limited.

HIV/AIDS counselling

It would be wrong to think in terms of HIV/AIDS counselling as an identifiable package. There are many special aspects that will be appropriate for some individuals but not all, e.g. sexual counselling, health counselling, drug counselling, bereavement counselling, contraception and abortion, adoption, and so forth. Moreover there are some special situations, e.g. prisons, occupational health, that will require specialist knowledge.

Broadly the aims of HIV counselling may be understood as those that apply to any counselling which may be variously defined as helping people to make decisions about their lives, supporting people through periods of difficulty or adjustment, etc. (see Chapter 1). However the specific objectives of a particular counselling situation will depend crucially upon the individual's health status, social relationships and the situation of their physical lives. Several possible objectives can be identified:

- to help those persons with AIDS
- to support and protect the health of those with HIV infection
- to advise those at risk of HIV to avoid danger to their own health
- to advise those with HIV upon the minimization of risk of transmission to others
- to support the carers of those with AIDS
- to help those with irrational fears about AIDS
- to support those professionals working within HIV/AIDS contexts.

Counselling practices for these different objectives will also differ. For example, supporting the carers of someone with AIDS may involve counselling for anxiety management or preparation for future bereavement. By contrast, advising upon risk reduction may be concerned more with behaviour modification. It is essential that principles of good practice for HIV counselling are widely disseminated (Bond, 1991).

One important area for counselling in relation to AIDS concerns counselling and HIV testing. Diagnostic HIV tests have been available in the UK since 1985 and are available on demand. Many people see testing as an effective means of combatting AIDS despite its limitations as a personal precaution. It must be recognized, however, that there are disadvantages as well as advantages attached to taking the test and counselling is necessary pre-test and if the person takes the test, post-test as well (McCreaner, 1989).

Someone wishing to take an HIV test must be fully informed about the implications whether the outcome is positive or not, and should have the opportunity to consider the risks to themselves before taking the test. There are possible legal, financial and occupational implications as well as social ones that may affect relationships with family, friends and lovers. In addition they should be advised upon risk reduction if it seems that their behaviour places them at risk of HIV infection. Among those requesting a test will be the 'worried well', i.e. individuals who have an excessive and unrealistic concern about HIV infection when they are at little risk of past, present or future infection. They also need pre-test counselling and may require information about the transmission of HIV. Despite any reassurances about their limited risk some will decide to take the test and will require further counselling despite the high probability of a negative test result.

Whatever the outcome of an HIV test, post-test counselling is essential. A negative result may still demand that a person be given advice about risks. Simply taking the test may have value to a person, causing them to assess the risk of their current behaviours. Of course, a positive result may lead to crisis, and post-test counselling following a positive outcome must try to achieve many different goals, e.g. advice upon sexual relationships including information upon safer sex, advice upon telling and talking to others, including sexual partners past and future as well as current partners. Clients may also wish to discuss their own needs for counselling and social support, and their arrangements for positive health care, as well as practical issues that may arise such as housing or childcare.

Counselling people with AIDS

The diagnosis of AIDS is traumatic for the patient and those who care for them. The social representation of AIDS emphasizes its fatality and its associations with prejudice and stigmatization cause further concerns. The person with AIDS and their family and friends will need help to adjust to the new situation and to their emotional reactions.

From the predicted increases in AIDS cases and their economic cost, it is increasingly likely that people with AIDS will be cared for in the community rather than in hospital. Those with AIDS may also wish this. If it is the case informal care from relatives, friends and lovers will need supplementing with adequate support services in the community for those infected *and* the carers. This will involve community welfare services whose personnel may require additional training if the necessary infrastructure is to be developed to support those with AIDS (Samuel and Boyle, 1989). It is essential that community policies and practices offer an integrated and complementary service to meet the differing needs of the many people who will experience the consequences of the diagnosis of AIDS – mothers, pregnant women, children, haemophiliacs, etc. (see particularly Green and McCreaner, 1989).

POSTSCRIPT

The social behaviours by which HIV is transmitted are complex and the interventions to limit the further spread of AIDS that are found to be effective for one community or culture may not be applicable to others. The issues of some developing countries may differ from those faced by the major industrial nations. It follows that the most practical emphasis for health practitioners will be the development of *local* strategies against AIDS. There is evidence, particularly from initiatives in the USA, that local community-based actions can be effective in the primary prevention of AIDS. For example, community-based outreach programmes in which injecting drug users are taught how to sterilize injecting equipment can reduce the risk of HIV infection in the local community (Watters, 1989).

It is widely acknowledged that mass media campaigns encouraging changes in sexual behaviour such as using condoms or restricting the number of sexual partners have not brought about significant changes in behaviour. However, community initiatives for gay men based upon peer-led prevention campaigns have produced encouraging reductions in risk behaviours (Kelly *et al.*, 1991). The same approach which uses socially influential individuals in a local community to endorse risk reduction could be equally useful for others including young adolescents and adult heterosexuals. These and other interventions must be evaluated if we are to determine the most effective strategies for achieving behavioural change.

Similar arguments apply to HIV counselling. Despite its widespread use there have been few attempts to evaluate its effectiveness. Few studies have sought to measure the impact of counselling on any aspect of clients' behaviours, their well-being, attitudes or health. Much research is urgently needed in this area to optimize the provision of counselling for both risk reduction and management of AIDS.

CONCLUSION

Caring for persons with AIDS and those who care for them is an immediate priority for workers in health care organizations. It will remain so for many years to come as the AIDS epidemic has yet to peak. Longer term, the solution must be primary prevention of HIV infection. That will require an orchestrated response involving international cooperation, national policies, and local interventions for community groups. Health professionals, welfare workers, counsellors and other practitioners will be involved in these responses at all levels. It is essential that their training should reflect this.

REFERENCES

Bond, T. (1991) *HIV Counselling*, Report on National Survey and Consultation 1990, British Association for Counselling/Department of Health, London

Coates, T.J. (1990) Strategies for modifying sexual behaviour for primary and secondary prevention of HIV disease, *Journal of Consulting and Clinical Psychology*, **58**, 57–69.

Green, J. (1989) Counselling for HIV infection and AIDS: the past and the future, *AIDS Care*, **1**, 5–10.

Green, J. and McCreaner, A. (eds.) (1989) *Counselling in HIV Infection and AIDS*, Blackwell Scientific Publications, Oxford.

Kelly, J.A., St Lawrence, J.S., Diaz, Y.E. *et al*. (1991) HIV risk behaviour reduction following intervention with key opinion leaders of a population: an experimental community-level analysis, *American Journal of Public Health*, **81**, 168–71.

McCreaner, A. (1989) Pre-test counselling, In J. Green and A. McCreaner (1989), above.

Melton, G. (1988) Adolescents and prevention of AIDS, *Professional Psychology: Research and Practice*, **19**, 403–8.

Mulleady, G.M., White, D.G., Phillips, K.C. and Cupitt, C. (1990) Reducing sexual transmission of HIV for injecting drug users: The challenge for counselling, *Counselling Psychology Quarterly*, **3**, 325–41.

Phillips, K.C. (1991) The primary prevention of AIDS, In M.K. Pitts and K.C. Phillips (eds.) *The Psychology of Health: An introduction*, Routledge, London.

Samuel, J.C. and Boyle, M. (1989) AIDS training and Social Services, *AIDS Care*, **1**, 287–96.

Schilling, R.F., El-Bassel, N., Schinke, S.P., Gordon, K. and Nichols, S. (1991) Reducing sexual transmission of AIDS: Skills building with recovering female drug users, *Public Health Reports*, **106**, 297-304

Watters, J.K. (1989) Observations of the importance of social context in HIV transmission among intravenous drug users, *Journal of Drug Issues*, **19**, 9–26.

White, D.G., Phillips, K.C., Clifford, B.R., Davies, M., Elliott, J.R. and Pitts, M.K. (1989) AIDS and intimate relationships: Adolescents' knowledge and attitudes, *Current Psychology: Research and Reviews*, **8**, 130–43.

14

Children in court

Julian Boon, Graham Davies and Elizabeth Noon

The last few years have seen a surge of interest in children's evidence, both from professionals who work with the increasing number of children who are involved in court proceedings, and also from the public in the wake of highly publicized enquiries such as those conducted at Cleveland and Orkney. This sharpened focus has provided the impetus for a mood of review which in turn has led to procedural changes in the rules for taking children's evidence. Currently rules for taking evidence from children vary widely from country to country. In some countries children as young as three years old have been permitted to give evidence while in others, children are prevented from giving evidence on the basis of age. Up until the Criminal Justice Act 1991, English case law made it very difficult to call children under eight years to give evidence. As Flin and Boon (1988) noted, this was unfortunate because children of this age were not too young to be victims of sexual assault, and were able to give a coherent account of the events in question.

As a result of recent changes in thinking in a number of countries, children may now be more readily heard (see Spencer *et al.*, 1989, for a review). However, it is far from clear whether the court room is an appropriate environment for eliciting the most accurate and helpful evidence from children. In this chapter we consider broader issues, including the ability of children to cope as witnesses, how best to prepare and help them before, during and after giving evidence, and recent procedural innovations designed to help the child witness.

The legal system of Great Britain (and likewise other countries such as Canada, America, Australia, etc., which are derived from the British system) is operated within an 'adversarial' framework. Essentially, under such a system, trials represent a contest in which the prosecution presents its case against the accused and the defence seeks to undermine and discredit it. It is the court which ultimately decides whether or not the prosecution has proved its case. This system contrasts with the 'inquisitorial' approach adopted in Germany (Frehsee, 1989) and other European countries where the court conducts its own enquiry in order to establish the truth. Such a system appears to facilitate the hearing of child witnesses (McEwan, 1988) but much can be done by effective preparation to empower child witnesses within the adversarial system.

Hitherto, the bulk of research has concentrated on children's abilities to recall information under laboratory conditions and has seldom considered their perceptions of the court, its physical characteristics, its functions, and the abilities of court practitioners to elicit accurate testimony. Furthermore, it is only very recently that researchers have focused their attention on how children cope with the experience of giving evidence (Flin *et al.*, 1990; Goodman *et al.*, in press; Morgan and Plotnikoff, 1989). It is of the utmost importance to establish what children understand about courts and procedures since this will play a correspondingly important part in their experiences and behaviour as witnesses. In addition, since the various legal practitioners play a critical role in determining what happens to children when they go to court, it is important to know how they in turn perceive the position of child witnesses. This research is reviewed in the following section.

CHILDREN'S PERCEPTIONS OF COURTS AND COURT PROCESSES

Research has been conducted in Britain and America surveying professionals (including social workers, police, prosecutors and judges) who have experience with working with child witnesses to establish what they felt caused stress to children (Flin *et al.*, 1988; Whitcomb *et al.*, 1985). The findings indicated several key problem areas: fear of cross-examination, unfamiliarity with the formalities of court, waiting in court and postponements, and having to give evidence in front of the accused. In addition, references were made to the unsuitability of the court design (e.g. the raised seating of judges, chair sizes, the isolation of the witness box), the extensive size of courtrooms and their generally poor acoustic properties. As part of the same Scottish study, Flin *et al.* asked children who were waiting to give evidence how they felt and the majority reported they were scared or worried. When these researchers asked why, the children tended to confirm the views of the professionals. Among fears reported were: retribution and being in the presence of the accused, not understanding what would be expected of them, being unable to recall the incident well enough, being on their own in the witness box, and speaking out in the courtroom.

Children's knowledge of the courts and their processes has been investigated by a number of researchers (Cashmore and Bussey, 1989; Flin *et al.*, 1989; Warren-Leubecker *et al.*, 1989). All of these studies showed that while children's knowledge improves with age, children of 6–7 years have a negligible grasp of the concept of a court and its processes. This has particularly serious ramifications for children's behaviour in court since the younger children often had unpleasant if not sinister misconceptions of courts and their processes. For example, Spencer and Flin (1990) report that a consistent misconception of an individual being prosecuted was that he or she would be 'badly hurt', 'hung', 'killed', or 'jailed'. It is very difficult to believe that such misapprehensions could have anything other than a stressful and inhibiting effect on a young witness giving evidence.

Furthermore, as will be noted below, fear of the unknown may intimidate children into recanting evidence, resulting in still greater pressure being placed upon them when in the courtroom.

In a bid to attenuate this fear of the unknown and dispel dangerous misconceptions, a number of agencies in Britain (West Yorkshire Police, Children's Legal Centre) have begun to make available leaflets and booklets to child witnesses and their parents which are intended to provide a clearer picture of what will happen (see also Bray, 1988, for an excellent book written by a social worker for use with very young children). However, leaflets are unlikely to provide a comprehensive answer.

In one study carried out in Scotland, Boon and Knox (1991) first established that a group of seven year old children had little or no idea about courts. Subsequently, these children read with their carers an explanatory booklet currently sent out with citations to appear in court; but when re-tested afterwards, no significant benefit to their understanding was found and in some instances confusion resulted. For another group of ten year old children, however, who had already some knowledge about courts and their purpose, the booklet was found to be of benefit. It is therefore particularly important that information be relevant to the age and characteristics of the witnesses concerned. In North America and Australia a wide and flexible range of materials is available to help explain the courts and their processes and this flexible approach is imperative if young children are to be genuinely helped and prepared to give evidence effectively.

There are many other ways of helping children give of their best and the majority of these techniques are known to legal practitioners. However, in our experience they are not applied consistently to all children, not even within the same trial. In the next section we consider these techniques and emphasize ways of maximizing their benefit to children.

PREPARING THE CHILD FOR COURT

In our experience it is particularly useful to arrange visits to show children an example of a courtroom when it is empty and free from threat. At this visit it can be explained who will be sitting where and even allow children to try their various chairs. Where this has been done we have seen children transformed from appearing extremely nervous and in awe of their surroundings to being comfortable and able to converse in a confident way. This is also a very useful opportunity to consolidate and integrate what may have been said before to children about what is expected of them (e.g. speaking the truth, saying if they don't understand, etc.) within the courtroom itself.

It is important for the person looking after the child to minimize the impression that the accused will be or even may be punished – such suggestions create expectations that may be neither welcome to the child nor fulfilled by the court. To the extent that purpose-related explanations of the court's function are required, relatively neutral alternatives such as 'to hear what everyone has to say' are preferable. For a variety of reasons, punishment orientations could increase the stress on children and inhibit their willingness to answer questions. These include: an increased sense of the fear of retribution; concern that they will be getting someone into trouble (especially where acquaintances and relatives are involved); and the related implication that the court is to do with frightening and unpleasant consequences. In addition, children could become upset if the accused is acquitted which can lead to feelings of being let down or disbelieved. The best orientation would seem to introduce the court as a place where people go to tell the truth and say what happened.

If someone other than the social worker arranging the court visit is bringing the child to the court on the day of the trial, it is very helpful to explain to them and the child the need to bring toys, games or books to help pass the time while waiting. This can be a very trying and stressful time for accompanying adults, children and court staff alike, especially as children can frequently wait all day or even longer to give evidence. In a large scale study in which researchers observed 89 child witnesses in Glasgow, more than a third gave their evidence a day or more later than they had been cited to attend court (Flin *et al.*, 1990). The importance of keeping children amused over such long delays and of maintaining good relations with the court staff can prove critical. An example of this was observed by the first author where a tired and bored seven year old boy was threatened by an exasperated court officer with being put in the cells if he could not be quiet. The resultant extreme distress resulted directly in the child not giving evidence and played a major part in the abandonment of the trial.

In addition, it is very helpful to be familiar with the layout of the court buildings – especially in areas where children may come into contact with the accused or witnesses for the defence. Such meetings can occur at any time while going to court and waiting to give evidence. If at all possible, side doors and separate waiting rooms should be found, and alternative travel facilities arranged. It is also worth exploring the possibilities of alternative catering facilities since witnesses for the defence, or even the accused who may be bailed over lunchtime, are likely to use the same court restaurant. Although a failure to isolate

the child from stress-evoking individuals can and does occur
by accident, it can occur by design as well. One such example
is cited by Joyce Plotnikoff (1989):

> 'A child left alone by the escorting social worker was told by
> her grandmother, "It will kill grandfather (the defendant) if
> you give evidence."'

Such pernicious interventions underline the need for both constant supervision and careful preparation in such matters as
locating suitable and safe waiting rooms.

A number of means of reducing the formality of the court are
available including: the removal of wigs and/or gowns; clear-
ance of the public from the court; the judge conducting examinations from the well of the court; the child being interviewed
at the Clerk or 'lawyers' table; parents/supporters being allowed to sit near the child; the child sitting with the judge on
the Bench; the child being allowed to sit as opposed to stand in
the witness box; microphones to amplify the child's voice,
especially when recounting stressful details; and the use of
screens to allow the child to give evidence away from the direct
gaze of the accused. All of these would seem to be sensible
measures to minimize the alien nature of the court and its
members, yet their implementation seems to be unpredictable
and more dependent on an individual judge's views than any
coherent set of rules or guidelines. This is also unfortunate
because it makes it that much harder to prepare the child
accurately for what he or she may expect. If it is possible to
speak to the prosecutor beforehand, then a request can be made
before the child enters the courtroom to implement at least
some of these arrangements. Local liaison with the Crown
Prosecution Service in England and Wales or the Fiscal's service
in Scotland will determine how easy it is for the supporter or
social worker to obtain access to the prosecutor to make the
necessary arrangements.

For children too, it is not normally possible to meet counsel
in Crown Court trials prior to their court appearance. In the
USA, as in England and Wales, it is not usual for witnesses to
meet prosecuting counsel before trial, a situation similar to that
in Scotland where the prosecuting counsel (known as the Ad-
vocate Depute) does not meet witnesses. However, in general
such meetings are not precluded by the code of conduct for

counsel and some do make an effort to make contact. In the lower courts it is possible for the prosecuting lawyer to meet the child beforehand; however, in our experience there is seldom enough time for such a meeting to occur. This means that in most cases the child is initially examined by a complete stranger with accompanying problems for establishing rapport. Furthermore, this problem is compounded by the genuine difficulties encountered by highly articulate lawyers, who are steeped in legal jargon, in communicating with children in court.

We have seen numerous instances where children have become confused by standard legal terminology (e.g. 'If your lordship pleases', 'My learned friend earlier asked', 'This might be a suitable moment for adjournment'). In questioning, too, difficulties in adopting sufficiently simple phraseology and language (e.g. double negatives – 'Did you not earlier say you had not done so?' – or unfamiliar phrases – 'What is your position regarding...', 'Did he take offence?') may result in a breakdown in communication.

The implications of this for the preparation of children are that they should be encouraged as much as possible to say if they do not understand the questions and be assured that no-one will be angry if they do so. Arguably a more effective preventive measure would be the provision of some form of skills and awareness training for lawyers who deal with children – something which, encouragingly, many lawyers have told us they would welcome.

EXAMINATION AND CROSS-EXAMINATION

All of the above measures for preparing and looking after children before court are of value in helping them deliver their evidence in as composed and clear a way as possible. However, the experience of being interrogated in court is still daunting for children as well as adults. In the Glasgow study, more than half of the 89 children observed were judged as being tense (57%) and unhappy (55%) during the initial examination carried out by the prosecution (Flin *et al.*, 1990). However, although it has frequently been claimed that the cross-examination is the most stressful part of the courtroom appearance and when the child will be most vulnerable to pressure from unscrupulous defence lawyers (e.g. Brennan and Brennan, 1990), this does not always appear to be the case. Indeed, defence lawyers have claimed that they would not be wise to put children under undue pressure for fear of losing the sympathy of the judge and jury.

Furthermore, the very nature of the adversarial system makes this unlikely. It is intended, during the initial examination-in-chief, that the prosecuting lawyer obtains from the child witness the facts that he or she knows about the alleged crime. If at this time the witness recants or shows reticence in reiterating what he or she is alleged to have said before in statements, the prosecution often has to meet that resistance in order to get the witness to reiterate the points in court. This can involve considerable stress for the witness who may well be afraid to speak in front of a known accused, while at the same time under strong pressure from the prosecuting lawyer to do so.

Thereafter, the defence's right to cross-examine will almost certainly be exercised if the witness has said anything which incriminates his client. It is at this point that the child is likely to be asked questions which attempt to undermine and discredit the initial examination-in-chief. Typical approaches include 'I put it to you that you have not told the truth'. If the child yields to this sort of pressure by recanting or acknowledging the possibility that the evidence given earlier may have been incorrect, it will almost certainly result in a second examination by the prosecution. In this instance the prosecuting lawyer's task is to encourage the witness to re-affirm the incriminating sections of the examination-in-chief, which in serious cases means yet again going over the unpleasant details under pressure.

In the Glasgow study, ratings were made for the degree of supportiveness that the lawyers showed towards the child when conducting their examinations. The findings fitted with these interpretations, showing that while the prosecution lawyers were more supportive during the examination-in-chief than were the defence lawyers during their cross-examination, this difference disappeared when they conducted their re-examinations. Complementing this, it was found that these trends were accompanied by significant reductions in the confidence that the children showed in their statements during cross-examination and re-examination relative to examination-in-chief.

Furthermore, it also should be noted that not all children are cross-examined only once. Where a case concerns more than one accused, each defence lawyer may require to cross-examine the witness. In one murder trial seen by the first author this involved no less than eight cross-examinations – ten examinations overall including the two from the prosecution. Cases such as this have done much to speed up the introduction of technological innovations designed to facilitate the production and presentation of children's evidence and these are described in the final section.

TECHNOLOGICAL INNOVATIONS IN COURTROOM PROCEDURE

The courts in England and Wales have in recent years introduced major technical innovations designed to ease the plight of children giving evidence in criminal proceedings involving sexual or physical violence: the live videolink and pre-recorded videotaped interviews respectively.

The function of the videolink is to enable a child to give evidence and be examined without ever seeing the accused or having to enter the courtroom. The child sits in a small room adjacent to the courtroom with an adult supporter whose function is purely to entertain the child and provide supervision when evidence is not being given. The supporter can be a police officer or social worker who is known to the child or even a complete stranger, the choice is entirely within the discretion of the individual judge. No person called as a witness can act as a supporter. The child sits in front of a workstation: a device the size of a domestic television set which contains a screen and a camera. Similar workstations are available to the judge and to the defence and prosecution lawyers sitting in court. In addition, television monitors are set up in the courtroom for the benefit of the jury, the accused and the public. The television circuit is set up in such a way as the child sees and hears whoever is talking to them at the time while those in court always see the child. In addition, judges have a 'panic button' which enables them to switch off the child's screen in the event of a legal objection during evidence or an outburst from the dock.

In England and Wales, the use of the videolink is at the discretion of the judge on application from counsel and is restricted to witnesses under 14 years in cases of physical violence and 17 years in cases of sexual assault. The videolink is currently available in some 24 courts and legislation now permits its use in Scotland. A survey by Davies and Noon (1991) revealed widespread acceptance of the link by both judges and barristers. The main perceived advantages of the link were that it enabled children to provide a more complete account of their evidence at trial and that children were more composed and less visibly distressed by the experience. A minority expressed residual concerns that the link might hinder the establishment of rapport with children or reduce the impact of their evidence in the eyes of the jury. Nevertheless in the first two years of use, some 544 cases had gone ahead with the aid of the link and its continuing use in the court seems assured.

Videolinks are also in regular use in some Australian states, notably Australian Capital Territories, and in New Zealand. Their use was first pioneered in the United States, but the employment of links has been curtailed by a Supreme Court decision that they violate the 'confrontation requirement' embodied in the US Constitution which guarantees the right of the accused to confront witnesses at trial. It is necessary to demonstrate that the child will be adversely affected by sight of the accused before such procedure can be invoked. The same applies to the second technological innovation: the use of pre-recorded videotaped interviews as a substitute for the child's live appearance for examination-in-chief in the courtroom.

Under the scheme now law in England and Wales, such tapes will comprise formal interviews typically conducted by a team made up of a social worker and a police officer who will receive special training for the task. Before such tapes may be shown in the court they will be viewed by the judge who will decide whether the style of questioning and the content are sufficiently compatible with the rules of evidence to be acceptable to the court. A code of practice on the conduct of such interviews has been drawn up by the Home Office and interviews will be expected to adhere to this as far as possible. It is hoped that the introduction of such tapes will enable a record to be obtained of the evidence soon after a child's original complaint, ensuring a full, spontaneous statement, unmarred by the impact of procedural delay and repeated questioning. Further, the child should be spared examination-in-chief in court, though cross-examination will continue to take place at trial, albeit normally on the videolink.

The Pigot Report (1989), on which these latter procedures are based, recommended that both prosecution examinations and cross-examinations should take place outside court and be recorded on tape, but the recommendation regarding cross-examination was not accepted. It remains to be seen whether the present 'half way house' provides an acceptable compromise.

In the meantime, children in England and Wales and other countries which practise the adversarial system will continue to require effective preparation for court. We have tried to point out practical suggestions for helping children present their evidence in the least stressed, least fragmented and most accurate ways. In our view their adoption would enhance standards of justice for both the witness and the accused, with better evidence and a greater likelihood of correctly convicting the guilty and acquitting the innocent.

REFERENCES

Boon, J.C.W. and Knox, A. (1991) Courting problems? An evaluation of one attempt to prepare children to give evidence, unpublished manuscript, Glasgow College, Scotland.

Bray, M. (1988) *Suzie and the Wise Hedgehog Go to Court*, Hawkesmere, London.

Brennan, M. and Brennan R. (1990) *Strange Language*, 3rd edn, Riverina Murray Institute of Higher Education, Wagga Wagga.

Cashmore, J. and Bussey, K. (1989) Children's conceptions of the witness role, in J. Spencer, G. Nicholson, R. Flin and R. Bull (eds.) *Children's Evidence in Legal Proceedings*, Faculty of Law, University of Cambridge, Cambridge.

Davies, G.M. and Noon, E. (1991) *An Evaluation of the Live Link for Child Witnesses* , The Home Office, London.

Flin, R. and Boon, J.C.W. (1988) The child witness in court, in C. Wattam, J. Hughes, and H. Blagg (eds.) *Child Sexual Abuse*, Longman, London.

Flin, R., Bull, R., Boon, J.C.W. and Knox, A. (1990) *Child Witnesses in Criminal Prosecutions*, Final Report to The Scottish Home and Health Department, Aberdeen.

Flin, R., Davies, G.M. and Tarrant, A. (1988) *The Child Witness*, Final Report to the Scottish Home and Health Department, Aberdeen.

Flin, R., Stephenson, Y. and Davies, G.M. (1989) Children's knowledge of court proceedings, *British Journal of Psychology*, **80**, 285–97.

Frehsee, D. (1989) Children's evidence within the German legal system, in J. Spencer, G. Nicholson, R. Flin and R. Bull (eds.) *Children's*

Evidence in Legal Proceedings, Faculty of Law, University of Cambridge, Cambridge.

Goodman, G., Taub, E., Jones, D., *et al.* (in press) Emotional effects of criminal court testimony on child sexual assault victims, *Monographs of the Society for Child Development*.

McEwan, J. (1988) Child evidence: More proposals for reform, *Criminal Law Review*, 813–22.

Morgan, J. and Plotnikoff, J. (1989) Children as victims of crime: Procedure at court, in J. Spencer, G. Nicholson, R. Flin and R. Bull (eds.) *Children's Evidence in Legal Proceedings*, Faculty of Law, University of Cambridge, Cambridge.

Pigot, Judge T. (1989) *Report of the Advisory Group on Video Evidence*, HMSO, London.

Plotnikoff, J. (1989) *The Child Witness*, Children's Legal Centre, London.

Spencer, J.R. and Flin, R.F. (1990) *The Evidence of Children: The law and the psychology*, Blackstone, London.

Spencer, J.R., Nicholson, G., Flin, R. and Bull, R. (eds.) (1989) *Children's Evidence in Legal Proceedings*, Faculty of Law, University of Cambridge, Cambridge.

Warren-Leubecker, A., Tate, C., Hinton, I. and Ozbeck, N. (1989) What do children know about the legal system and when do they know it? In S. Ceci, D. Ross and M. Toglia (eds.) *Perspectives on Children's Testimony*, Springer, New York.

Whitcomb, D., Shapiro, E.R. and Stellwagen, C.D. (1985) *When the Victim is a Child: Issues for judges and prosecutors*, National Institute of Justice, Washington DC.

Section Four

Practitioners and Research

15

Making use of research

Chris Lewis

WHAT IS RESEARCH?

'Research' is arguably one of the most loaded words in the English language, a convenient way of raising the intellectual status of many of our common activities. 'I think I'll go and find out how much houses are in the area' sounds far less impressive than 'I think I'll go and research the housing market in the area'. 'My children have gone to the library to find out where fossil fuels come from' may be far less awe-inspiring than, 'My children have gone to the library to research the origins of fossil fuels'. 'I really would like to understand more about eating disorders' may have less impact than, 'I really should become familiar with the research on eating disorders'. Each of these statements substitutes 'research' for either 'finding out' or 'understanding'. Is this fair? Is this all that 'research' means?

Leedy (1989) argues that it is essential to distinguish between 'research' and 'true research'. The first is meaningless jargon; the second can be identified with seven distinct characteristics:

1. Research originates with a question
2. Research demands a clear articulation of a goal
3. Research requires a specific plan or procedure
4. Research usually divides the principal problem into more manageable sub-problems
5. Research is tentatively guided by constructs called 'hypotheses'
6. Research will count only hard, measurable data in attempts to resolve the problem that initiated the research
7. Research is, by its nature, circular or, more exactly, helical.

What Leedy is really trying to say here is that true research must be distinguished from mere information-gathering and rummaging for information; therefore research is more than just finding out or understanding. This view, however, can be set aside as all it is really saying is that true research requires that the researcher goes through a number of stages both consciously and systematically. This of course does not mean that in other sorts of research a procedure is not also followed, albeit less rigorously and below the threshold of awareness of the person conducting it. The person wishing to become more familiar with research on eating disorders, or indeed the child researching the origin of fossil fuels in the library, may well go through those stages.

If we consider these in order, it is hard to imagine that in either of these examples there would not be a question, very early on in the process, originating in the mind of the researcher. Both would possess the desirable level of inquisitiveness which is essential as a starting point to research. It is also quite likely that there is a clear articulation of the goal. It might be a statement from a teacher that has fuelled the enthusiasm in the child and sent them to the library in the first place. As far as a specific plan of procedure existing, quite clearly there will be an enormous range of sophistication in 'finding out' and 'understanding' the projects referred to in our example. Indeed the range is as large, perhaps, as is found in what most would accept as true research.

Again, dividing the principal problem into sub-problems is, of course, a natural cognitive phase, gone through by almost anyone trying to understand anything. Once it is realized that the main problem is too large to cope with, it is inevitably subdivided into manageable bits. The logic that is applied to the ordering and handling of the bits is the sensible guide to efficiency in all research, as Leedy (1989) points out: 'Because many researchers take neither the time nor the trouble to isolate the lesser problems within the major problem, their research projects become cumbersome and unwieldy'. Thus with regard to this, is there a difference between the 'true researcher' and those who are just trying to 'find out'?

It is of course true that the feature of 'true research' is the existence of explicit hypotheses which gives direction to the research process, but maybe the difference is simply that in 'real research' hypotheses are stated as opposed to just being logical suppositions in the mind of the researcher. But in both cases hypotheses are being used. Indeed this is something we do in our everyday existence. Something is observed and we immediately need an explanation for why this has happened. We make guesses and we make assumptions, both as aids to increase our understanding. If we are prepared to delay the feeling that we have justified our guesses or validated our assumptions until we have collected more information then we have been 'hypothesizing'. Thus it can be argued that in any sort of research activity there will inevitably be a sequence of the development and testing of hypotheses.

It is reasonable to maintain that research will only countenance hard, measurable data in attempting to resolve problems, if the meanings of 'hard' and 'measurable' are carefully interpreted. Developments in the use of 'qualitative' methods (as discussed in Chapters 16 and 17) give a lie to the traditionally held view that these two concepts essentially require quantification. All that 'hardness' requires is quality of data; all that 'measurable' requires is an awareness of a change in the level of understanding. It is very likely that the child researching in the library will experience these.

Finally, the idea that 'true research' concludes with raising further problems which require investigating, thus setting the whole process off again, is obviously generalizable to less well structured 'finding out' procedures. It would be almost impossible for the child who has now learnt about the origins of fossil fuels not to be stimulated into further inquisitive activity, perhaps the likeliest of these being the attempt to regenerate the research cycle once more to answer the question 'So what?'. It would seem therefore not as easy as might at first be expected to identify a marked distinction between research and 'true research'. If there are any such distinctions, they exist only in the realms of planning and formality.

What is the relevance of the above debate, therefore, to those in the health professions? First and foremost, it is that the label 'research' can be applied to a very wide range of activities that many workers in the field undertake on a day-to-day basis. For that reason it should be recognized and valued. It is not simply an ivory-tower activity, participation in which requires membership of some elite academic club. The pursuit of just trying to 'find out' can still produce rich information. To set out to research the level of job satisfaction amongst nurses working in a geriatric unit, it could well be wise to consider the use of well-drafted and extensive questionnaires, highly structured interviews and carefully monitored in-depth group discussions, but one could go some way down the road in matching the results of these methods by simply asking the nursing staff two questions: 'How satisfied are you with your work?' and 'Why do you feel like this?'.

In summary, the plea that is being made here is that research is something that all helping professionals can and should do on a day-to-day basis. What it requires is that what we learn from 'finding out' is catalogued and utilized. This would constitute the recognition of the importance of informal research. None of the above discussion, however, must be taken to lessen the importance of formal research and it is certainly true that many health professionals feel quite distanced from being allowed to comprehend this activity fully.

GETTING CLOSE TO FORMAL RESEARCH

In order to feel comfortable with formal research, it is important to appreciate firstly who are the researchers, what are research papers often trying to say and how can the published research best be used.

Who are the researchers?

Researchers in the field of applied psychology will largely be either academics or practitioners operating outside an academic environment. Also, researchers are predominantly white, middle class, male, heterosexuals and this may well determine a set of beliefs which the researcher identifies with. Researchers can therefore be criticized for operating from the premise that a particular group is the norm and, by definition, other groups will be seen as deviant or unusual in their behaviour. Meanwhile, supremacist conclusions are made or inferred about the group identified with.

Recent authors, for example, Spender (1980), Wilkinson (1986) and Kitzinger (1987), have noticed this phenomenon in relation to gender. Historically, females have been omitted from research with inferences being made regarding the behaviour of women from the findings on males. Recent attempts have sought to redress the balance but the focus has been on adding women into the research areas where they were previously overlooked. However feminist researchers are now challenging the fundamental assumptions on which research is based and the methodologies used, seeking to make a female perspective central to the research rather than an additional or comparative viewpoint. This challenge to the basis of hypotheses and conclusions encourages research to contribute to a broader understanding of the whole of human behaviour, not just specific groups or viewed from a particular perspective.

For those wishing to make use of research it is often useful to consider the motives of the researchers themselves. The pioneering spirit, the desire to push back 'the frontiers of human understanding' is real and is almost certain to be part of what underpins the researcher's efforts. But there are other motives. For academics, their career success will almost definitely depend on it. The number and quality of research publications still remain the major criteria used in the selection of senior academic posts, and, at other levels, active researching is to be found as an explicit condition in contracts of employment. For the applied psychology practitioner, credibility can be enormously enhanced, which in turn may promote distinct commercial advantages, especially for those in self-employment. In short, published research is a way of getting known within the applied psychology community, and therefore fosters any advantages that that might bring.

How are research papers produced?

As the bulk of research is produced in journals or periodicals, it is essential at this stage to distinguish between refereed and non-refereed publications. If a researcher wishes to gain maximum credibility from their academic peers, they will endeavour to report their research findings in a refereed journal. These are so called because it is normally the researcher who takes the initiative and submits a paper to the editorial board of the journal who will then pass the draft manuscript to other known experts in the field and ask them to comment on the suitability or otherwise of this piece of work for publication. This is certainly not a rubber-stamping exercise; it is a significant hurdle at which as many as 80% or 90% of submitted research reports can fall, depending on the journal in question. Because of this process, which may include papers being sent back to the author for revision, there can be quite a long time lapse between completion of the research and publication. A two year delay is certainly not unusual.

Non-refereed journals and periodicals approach research papers rather differently. Here the initiative may come not from the researcher, but from the editor of the journal who may approach the researcher in order to persuade them to supply the publication with an article. Here there tends to be little or no refereeing process, except the normal editorial scrutiny. The length of time between completion of research and publication can be quite short, sometimes as little as a few weeks.

A characteristic which strongly distinguishes the refereed from the non-refereed journals is the layout of the actual article or paper. Whereas non-refereed journals will have an individual layout in line with their own house style and one which may be very different from other non-refereed journals, the refereed ones tend to adopt an almost standard layout.

In submitting papers to these it is essential that researchers/authors adhere to that layout in their draft. The standardized layout for refereed papers is likely to be as follows:

1. The formal title, which may be quite full to avoid ambiguity and almost certainly avoids any cryptic tendencies.
2. The name of the author, followed by the institution or business with which they are associated and which will be deemed to have some relationship to the actual research contained in the paper.
3. An abstract, which, in a single paragraph normally not exceeding around 150 words, offers a description of the research design, method of analysis, results and major points from the discussion.
4. Introduction and review of the literature. The author should introduce the topic to the reader by describing major aspects of the body of knowledge on which they are basing their research. This part of the paper normally makes heavy use of references to other research, carefully quoting the author and year of publication of the research as the introduction unfolds. Ideally, this introductory review should crescendo at the point where the body of knowledge is crying out for an additional piece of research information, a gap which this very paper is

going, to some degree, to fill. This point may well be expressed in the form of explicitly identified hypotheses under investigation in this study.

5. Methodology. The way in which the research is to be conducted is now explained in detail. This includes the actual methodological procedure, the actual investigative methods and measures and indeed, the subjects on whom these measures are to be applied. It would probably not be libellous to say that most researchers do cheat a little at this point. The methodology should be an expression of that which is necessary to investigate the hypotheses which form the focus of the study. However, for much research the methodology that you actually want to use, especially in relation to subjects, might not be available quite as you would have wished when it comes to pursuing the project. As research papers, of course, are written after the event, there is a tendency to justify the actual methodological detail that was used rather than to explain the real short-fall from the original design. This should not be seen as a major criticism of the researchers as any reported methodology must at least be deemed as adequate.

6. Analysis of results. Here the methods of analysing the data are introduced and justified and indeed the contents of that analysis are presented. The traditional use of quantitative methods by applied psychologists means that this section normally contains examples of the application of statistical methods. Whilst in non-refereed journals there is often a tendency for authors to be discouraged from quoting the results of statistical analysis, or if they do, to do it with extreme simplicity, refereed journals will assume that the readers are familiar with statistical methods. This means that results sections are normally concerned to provide information that meets statistical conventions rather than to exhibit any notion of reader-friendliness. It is for this very reason that most professional training programmes that contain a heavy emphasis on applied psychology insist that students follow a course in statistics. Students have to be given the skills and knowledge to read research papers of this kind.

7. Discussion. With the results of this research producing data that can now be overlaid on the body of knowledge that was

reviewed in the introduction, it is now possible to discuss the implications of this additional information. It is at this point in the research paper that one perceives for the first time evidence of the researchers freeing themselves from the shackles imposed by the standardized reporting procedures. Of course the discussion will contain categorical statements that can be well supported by the results of the study, but it also allows the 'flying of some kites'. The word 'maybe' is often seen to appear, as are the more formal expressions of 'It could reasonably be argued that the evidence suggests ...' or 'Whilst it is not completely clearcut, there is some evidence to suggest...'

It is the discussion which allows the authors to pull together the various strands that are necessary to justify their efforts on this occasion, and it is very useful for the reader. It is also an opportunity for the researchers to give themselves an escape route against criticism from their academic peers. The final paragraph of many research papers often quite explicitly claims that any research findings contained therein should not be considered to be conclusive, that before findings can be accepted as such there is a need for others to replicate the research, or more generally that this particular piece of research has simply pointed to the fact that more research is necessary.

8. References. It is a very strict rule in refereed journals that all authors and dates of research that are quoted in the body of the paper are fully listed in this final section. There are very strict conventions which determine the actual layout of references, conventions which, one has to say, prove to be of enormous benefit to readers who have to find research papers through the reference listings.

Despite the rigorous standardization required by refereed journals, researchers in the field of psychology often approach the task of writing their research papers from inappropriate positions. They have misconceptions about the nature of research papers, which were usefully described some time ago (Sternberg, 1977). The misconceptions are:

1. 'Writing the psychology paper is the most routine, least creative aspect of the scientific enterprise, requiring much time but little imagination.' Not true. The purpose of writing

the paper should not just be to communicate your thoughts but to help you form and organize them.

2. 'The important thing is what you say, not how you say it.' Not true. A badly presented idea leaves the reader in a quandary trying to understand whether it is the quality of the idea or simply its presentation which is at fault. It is also probably true that the most well-known psychologists are those that are among the best writers.

3. 'Longer papers are better papers, and more papers are better yet.' Not true. Whilst there is nothing wrong with long papers, there is if the length is used as a way of avoiding tight organization and clear writing. Alternatively, the temptation to divide research up into its component parts and publish each as a separate paper often exists. This meets the need of those writers who count publications but not those who read them.

4. 'The main purpose of a psychology paper is the presentation of facts, whether newly established (as in reports of experiments) or well established (as in literature reviews).' Not true. The goal of science is not the accumulation of facts. It is the diverse explanation of them. Papers should be guided by ideas and points of view, with facts being presented in the service of these.

5. 'The distinction between scientific writing on the one hand and advertising or propaganda on the other is that the purpose of scientific writing is to inform whereas the purpose of advertising or propaganda is to persuade.' Not true. When a psychologist writes a paper they have in effect a product to sell, i.e. their ideas about why certain phenomena exist. As such it may well be the only product on the market and so the 'consumers' might need to be persuaded to 'buy' it. Authors of research papers have a marketing responsibility.

6. 'A good way to gain acceptance of your theory is by refuting someone else's theory.' Not true. Unless your argument is absolutely watertight there is a very good chance that the case you make will increase enthusiasm for the theories you are attempting to refute.

7. 'Negative results that fail to support the researcher's hypothesis are every bit as valuable as positive results that do support the researcher's hypothesis.' Not true. Whilst one would hope that researchers are honest and therefore

report their 'losses' as well as their 'wins', nonetheless negative results are hard to find in refereed journals. The reason for this is that research is often only designed to explain positive results. Negative results, if they occur, become uninterpretable.

8. 'The logical development of ideas in a psychology paper reflects the historical development of ideas in the psychologist's head.' Not true. As mentioned above, the neat logic of standardized presentation is rarely as it really happens. The methodology section is written with hindsight of what actually happened rather than what was originally intended.

Thus in understanding how research papers are produced it is important to recognize that the idea that authors of refereed journal articles plan their research and predict their findings well in advance, often down to the last detail, is in practice questionable. The adherence to standardized layouts might well be a function of ritual as much as the realities of the research activity.

How do we judge the value of a research paper?

Again we can turn to Sternberg (1977) for identifying standards for evaluating psychology research papers deemed to have some noticeable merit. In summary:

- The desire that a paper contains one or more surprising results that nevertheless make sense in some theoretical context.
- The results presented in the paper are of major theoretical or practical significance.
- The ideas in the paper are new and exciting, perhaps presenting a new way of looking at an old problem.
- The interpretation of results is unambiguous.
- The paper integrates into a new, simpler framework data that had previously required a complex, possibly unwieldy framework.
- The paper contains a major debunking of previously held ideas.
- The paper presents an experiment with a particularly clever paradigm or experimental manipulation.

• The findings and theory presented in the paper are general ones.

Whilst these 'rules' for evaluation of papers in psychology are extremely useful, they are much more likely to be applied by those who referee articles for publication. Whilst it is useful for the general reader of research to bear these in mind, they will find it much more useful to apply a simpler evaluation criterion, namely the 'So what?' test. Despite the complex presentation of statistical data, the heavily referenced literature review and the lengthy, careful and articulate discussions, the actual contribution that any given research paper makes to the body of knowledge is often quite simple and surprisingly small. In applied psychology research, the practical significance is unlikely to take your breath away.

But all of this does not lessen the usefulness of the research. After assimilating the contents of a research paper, the reader asks the question 'So what?'. If they cannot readily think of an answer then the paper has failed the test. The author has, as we discussed above, failed to deal with the marketing aspect of their efforts. The reader should also be able to take a step back from the paper and ask the question, 'What is the researcher trying to say?'. Again it is a severe criticism if there is not a quick and fairly easy to understand answer. Good research papers are those that pass the 'So what?' test with a lot to spare.

GUIDELINES ON USING RESEARCH PAPERS

We can now address the situation of the health professional who wishes to make use of research by improving their understanding of some particular aspect of the field of applied psychology. It is important to recognize that publications that make reference to research or contain research papers tend to be a trade-off between rigour and comprehension. The more rigorous the paper, the less easily understood by the non-specialist/lay person it is likely to be, whereas those that are designed for that readership can sometimes demonstrate shortfalls in quality both of presentation of the research or indeed of the design of the research itself. Obviously this issue relates to the way you define the non-specialist/lay person. Many rigorous refereed psychology journals are aimed at the professional applied psychologist. Those journals therefore may well view the health professional as a non-specialist.

An early decision which those wanting to make use of the research must make is which of these roads they should go down. The non-refereed, easy to read, pathway where journals are explicitly written for the non-specialist, or the rigorous route where journals tend to be written for others in the field of the researchers. Whilst the obvious question may be 'Why not go down both?', the answer is that research information systems have a bad record at cross-referencing between these two levels of publication. Refereed journals rarely make reference to non-refereed publications and non-refereed articles are very selective in their use of references anyway.

If the decision is to focus on the easier end, then it is wise to direct effort at being familiar with the content of the technical publications explicitly aimed at the health professions with a careful eye firmly directed towards the daily and weekly national press. To explore research in this way can be a very hit and miss affair, because of the few available publicly accessible information systems covering this sector of publications. However information offices that exist within large companies, institutions, health authorities or professional bodies may well have developed local systems that are well worth examining when trying to investigate research in this way.

If the decision is made to go down the more rigorous path, then the disadvantages presented by the rigour may well be counterbalanced by the existence of more efficient information retrieval systems. A good starting point is always to use basic textbooks. If we consider the example of the health professional wishing to research post-traumatic stress disorders, then they could consult well-established textbooks on applied psychology, especially clinical psychology and health psychology, and start by looking up 'stress' in the index. This may well lead to some basic references in the relevant sectors in the book which can then be further investigated in a suitable library.

A major facility for those wishing to research refereed journals is the use of *Psychological Abstracts*, which is an annually produced publication that reproduces the abstracts from journals published in the area of psychology in the English language. These are then cross-indexed. Again, looking up 'stress' or indeed 'post-traumatic stress' in this index will direct the investigator to the abstracts of relevant papers.

Even more efficient than this system has been the development recently of computer-based research literature reviewing, probably the best known of which is PSYCLIT. This system, which is available in many libraries, especially those in universities and colleges, enables the investigator to feed in key words and a computer program will search through all English language abstracts and identify those that contain these key words. Thus, if the health professional indicates 'post-traumatic stress disorder', any refereed paper that dealt with that topic to such an extent that it would feature in the abstract section of the paper would be identified. The system can produce the full abstract and references. Using the abstract as a way of screening out the research papers which clearly may not be of interest to them, they can then seek out copies of the full research papers. Clearly each research paper itself will contain a comprehensive list of references relating to other research in the area. The whole topic could then open up to the investigator, who could then make their own judgement about how widely and how deeply they wished to pursue this interest.

CONCLUSION

In conclusion, what is being said in this chapter is that research is essentially about finding out and this may be done with varying degrees of rigour and enthusiasm. People get involved in research for all sorts of reasons, some which are about the general good, others for very personal gain and satisfaction. This is really of no consequence, because the end result is the production of a body of knowledge, albeit of inconsistent quality. But it all helps. Bad research is often better than no research at all, providing that its limitations are recognized. The health professional must never feel at all discouraged from attempting to do their own research or to improve their technical knowledge and competence, or indeed simply to satisfy their inquisitiveness by becoming familiar with the research of others. It is important to approach it systematically, remembering that researchers are only human. It can take you along an undulating path, being at times hard going and at others disappointingly simplistic, but may well lead to a network which intrigues.

REFERENCES

Kitzinger, C. (1987) *The Social Construction of Lesbianism*, Sage, London.
Leedy, P.D. (1989) *Practical Research, Planning and Design*, 4th edn, Macmillan, New York.
Spender, D. (1980) *Manmade Language*, Routledge, London.
Sternberg, R.J. (1977) *Writing the Psychology Paper*, Barron, New York.
Wilkinson, S. (ed.) (1986) *Feminist Social Psychology*, Open University Press, Milton Keynes.

16

Analysing discourse: qualitative research and the helping professions

Harriette Marshall

Discourse analysis refers to the analysis of spoken and written texts, including for example policy documents, interviews, newspaper accounts and group discussions. Attention is directed at the structure of discourse with concern for the possible consequences of the use of particular accounts. This chapter will examine the contribution that discourse analysis can make to research concerning health professionals. The aim is to outline the differences between discourse analysis and traditional attitudinal approaches to research, using a study of maternity care as an illustration. It is argued that there are important theoretical and practical implications to such research. Specifically, concern moves away from categorizing individuals into those with positive or negative attitudes, in this case to individualized care, with a view to using this information as a basis for selection criteria. Instead, the focus moves to an examination of the possibilities and constraints of the various discourses about individualized care available to and made use of by health carers. Practically this implies redirecting attention at training structures and policy documents to ensure that fully articulated discussions of good care for all are present and widely communicated.

RESEARCH ON MATERNITY CARE

Recent British policy documents set out one component of good health care as being individualized or person-centred care (ARM, 1986; RCM, 1987; UKCC, 1986). This carries over into the domain of maternity care. Research findings have shown that women gave the highest rating of satisfaction with maternity care when they felt they had been given personalized care, and shown they were valued as people (Shields, 1978). Related to this, it has been argued that it is important for health carers to respond to the values of the consumer and make the consumer an active partner in making decisions about health care (Morales-Mann, 1989). Where women perceive themselves as playing little part in decision-making in labour, their satisfaction decreased (Birch, 1982).

Recent research that has examined health carers' perceptions of their work reflects this emphasis on individualized care (Morales-Mann, 1989). A brief examination of research in this area illustrates that the sort of questions that psychologists have posed include identifying individuals with both positive and negative attitudes to personalized care (Todman and Jauncey, 1987). Other research is clearly related to this concern with individualized care, for example the attempts to measure 'empathic care' (frequently equated with the ability to care for the person as an individual) (Gould, 1990; Chapman, 1983) or attempts to determine aspects of the 'empathic personality' (Sparling and Jones, 1977).

TRADITIONAL RESEARCH

The most typical approach to attitude measurement is to devise a questionnaire which comprises a number of statements each defined by the researcher as embodying a positive or negative attitude to a topic, in this case individualized care. Individual health carers are then asked to indicate their response to each statement on a scale ranging from strongly agree to strongly disagree. The overall responses are then calculated and the respondent categorized as holding either a positive or negative attitude to individualized care.

There are a number of methodological and theoretical points to make about this traditional approach. Methodologically, it should be noted that respondents are constrained in their responses; they cannot choose more than one response to each question, nor can they explain or justify a particular response. Respondents are also limited by the researcher's choice of statements, which are usually a short sentence, with no context provided. The researcher's interpretation of each statement is assumed to be the same as that of the respondent and no opportunity for the respondent to qualify their interpretation is offered. Further, it is the researcher who decides whether each statement is defined as indicating either a positive or a negative attitude. It is not possible for the respondent to discuss the ways in which their responses might vary according to the specific context or in relation to, for example, ways in which their ideal practice is constrained by practicalities. Despite these restrictions, the respondent will be categorized using the researcher's definitions as being one sort of individual as compared to another; for example, as an individual with a positive or progressive attitude to patient care, or one with a negative attitude.

Theoretically, this approach uses the individual as the unit for analysis. The assumption is that consistency in response indicates an underlying attitude held by that individual. Using this approach, language, as used in questionnaires in the statements and responses, is seen as a means of getting at some underlying reality; in this example, as a means to identify an attitude, seen to exist within the individual's head.

DISCOURSE ANALYSIS

Discourse analysis takes a different starting point. Discourse analysts take a different perspective towards language from that adopted by attitudinal researchers, arguing that language is not merely a descriptive medium, producing a reflection of some underlying reality, but that language actively constructs what we understand to be 'reality'.

Discourse analysts further argue that the 'action' orientation of language is veiled by the use of non-contextualized materials, as, for example, in the restricted choice of responses offered in questionnaire statements. Therefore discourse analysts consider that methodologically it is important *not* to restrict participants' responses, but to consider extended segments of talk and the context in which the discussions are made. It is thought that when responses are not restricted, variability will emerge.

The following section uses extracts from interviews about maternity care carried out with health carers to illustrate comparisons made between traditional and discourse analytic approaches. It does not represent a discourse analysis in itself but aims to illustrate three main issues on which attitudinal and discourse analysts differ. First, the meaning of statements on attitude questionnaires; second, the importance of examining contextualized conceptualizations of good maternity care; and third, the assumption that participants can be categorized as holding unified, consistent attitudes.

BACKGROUND TO THE STUDY

The extracts below are selected from interviews with 15 health carers all of whom were taking courses to gain further health qualifications. The interviews comprised 18 questions which were broadly structured into four main sections. First, questions concerning various aspects of health carers' work; second, their characterization of good maternity care; third, discussions of how to provide good care in various contexts and in respect to various practices including childbirth, feeding, childrearing and discipline; and finally questions about providing care for mothers from different ethnic groups. (For a more detailed account see Marshall, 1992.)

ANALYTIC PROCEDURE

The procedure follows Potter and Wetherell (1987). The first aim is to identify recurrent patterns in the linguistic constructions, referred to here as linguistic repertoires. This entails reading and rereading through the transcripts and picking out terms and phrases which refer, in this case, to maternity care and good practice which illustrated either (1) similarities in terms of structure or content, or (2) differences in what was being said. Initially any extracts which appeared to be loosely connected to maternity care were taken out. This process was repeated several times, first placing extracts under broad head-ings, such as agreement with 'individualized care', disagreement with 'individualized care', alternative notions, e.g. 'informing the client of good practice'. Second, attention was given to how the constructions were being used and whether they seemed to serve the same function. In this sense discourse analysis goes beyond a simple content analysis to explore the ways in which the various repertoires are being used and their possible consequences. One main consideration here was to examine the relationship between the repertoires, for example where one served to complement or undermine another.

Instances where ... appears in the extract indicate that there is material omitted from the extract. Interviewers' questions are prefixed with *'Int'* to differentiate them from participants' responses.

Talking about good maternity care

In terms of characterizing good care, the repertoire of 'individualized care' or 'person-centred care', was used in the majority of the accounts. The following extracts illustrate the way in which good maternity care is characterized as comprising attention to the individual woman's needs and choices, with an attempt made to establish a relationship with the mother and act in a partnership with her.

Int: How would you characterize good practice?

Midwife 1: I would like to think my practice is individual and that it is a case of being there for the woman and whatever she particularly wants.

Health Visitor 5: When I first meet someone I start initiating my own relationship, and I always spend some time defining my role and how I work, I try to have more of a partnership sort of approach, which obviously gives them more responsibility. I think if you explain and if you build on that, putting the emphasis more on them, for most people it works quite well.

Midwife 3: I think with the introduction of individualized care now, each woman is viewed as an individual ... each woman is viewed as an individual and is given care appropriate to her needs.

Midwife 6: I think my approach has changed quite a lot, because we were taught to rather take over with the care of the mother, I suppose you could use the term matriarchal and that was perceived as being the right way, say, 20 or 30 years ago. When I trained the conduct of labour was very much the 'push dear, push'. The perception of how to give care has changed so much, we didn't use to realize that the mother wanted to be a partner and I think we have to be careful because she doesn't always, sometimes she wants to put herself in our hands. So good care is being sensitive to the wishes and the needs of the mother.

In the above extracts individualized care is seen as indicative of good maternity care. Individualized care is referred to explicitly in these extracts, described as being where the needs and choices of individual women are met by appropriate care. The relationship between carer and mother is described as being a partnership thus implying that good care involves allowing women as clients to make decisions rather than having these dictated by the carer. This is set out clearly in the final extract where good practice now is contrasted with good practice in the past, and the change characterized in terms of control moving from the midwife to a shared partnership, with midwives finding out and respecting each woman's choices and decisions.

There would seem to be an unambiguously positive response to individualized care expressed in all these extracts. Listening to each individual woman's choices and decisions and responding appropriately appears to be unequivocally supported here. These sorts of characterizations of good care equalling individualized care were used by the majority of carers in their accounts.

If the accounts are examined further it might be suggested that this positive response to individualized care would be reflected in discussions around specific practices. It is important at this point to compare these accounts in relation to questionnaire statements that have been used by attitudinal researchers to assess participants' responses to person-centred care. One example of an attitudinal scale which is directly comparable here is that of Todman and Jauncey (1987). This comprises 19 items to measure attitudes to aspects of obstetric practice. Statement number 4 on their scale reads, 'Midwives should be more willing to comply with women's requests for alternative delivery positions, e.g. squatting'. Agreement with this statement is taken to indicate a positive attitude to personalized care. Taking the carers' accounts to examine their discussions of 'alternative birthing positions', it should be possible to see whether the translation from responses to attitude statements to the identification of an underlying attitude is as straightforward as attitudinal researchers would suggest.

> *Midwife 6*: If mother wants to, hopefully, well yes, we certainly do meet her needs. Well, we've had water births in the unit and they haven't exactly happened, but mothers have wanted them. We got a sort of skip thing from the National Childbirth Trust in the labour ward and they have used it. But the two we had, one needed help and had to get out anyway and the other found it so hot that she climbed out and had it on the bed. It makes the labour ward like a sauna, everything dripping. But I suppose that's been a leap forward. When I started, the thought of a woman choosing to that extent would have been absolutely unheard of … But I think there are barriers. I've never delivered anybody in an alternative position because, well, if you call left lateral alternative, I have, but not squatting or anything like that. Again I'm aware of a split within myself, the idea I think is lovely but if I have to take the responsibility for doing it myself I might feel nervous and I know things like water births I have a little bit of a hang up about the idea, because for the midwife's sake, the risk of blood-borne diseases, if she's going to be dabbling her hands in water up to her elbows, okay, I know that something like HIV can't penetrate intact skin, but if water is going to get inside her gloves, then there could be risks.

There are a number of points to consider in examining this extract. First the meaning of 'alternative' is questioned in terms of the breadth of the definition. Attitude scales are put together with the assumption that the meaning of the statements are the same for all respondents. However, within the extract above, the midwife explores the definition of 'alternative' and produces varying definitions of meaning that could be placed on the statement. Clearly the definition of 'alternative' is not unambiguous; this participant questions whether 'left lateral' is seen as being 'alternative', also mentioning squatting and water births.

Second, this extract shows that when the context is examined variability emerges. While support for allowing women to choose is clearly voiced, and seen as 'lovely' and 'a leap forward' from previous practices, there is a tension throughout the account which the participant refers to directly as 'a split within myself'. She explains this split by drawing on various qualifications and considerations around 'alternative births' including personal nervousness and 'hang up' around alternative births, to nurses' safety and practical effects on the ward. Implicit in her discussion is the consideration of her own accountability if there were problems with the birth. Thus, throughout the account justifications are given for *not* always supporting a mother's choice. What this one extract illustrates is that when responses are not restricted and participants are allowed more than an 'agree or disagree' response, the contextualized responses provide the researcher with a complex organization of accounts including justifications and qualifications. In other words, the action-oriented nature of talk emerges.

This sort of variability in response is not unusual. Although only one extract is presented here many various alternative examples could have been used to illustrate the complexity of discussion in relation to the presence of fathers at births, home births and feeding practices, all items included on previous attitude scales (Todman and Jauncey, 1987).

This sort of variability also presents a problem for attitudinal researchers in that attitudes are taken to be stable across situations. The rationale behind such attitude scales is to identify people with negative attitudes to person-centred care, because these negative attitudes are thought to influence health carers' practice. Attitude researchers have acknowledged for some time now that the relationship between attitudes and behaviour is not straightforward and that behaviour is only partially influenced by attitudes (Fishbein and Azjen, 1975). Behaviour or practice is not a straightforward expression of an attitude but is shaped by numerous other variables. The emerging inconsistency in the attempt to identify an attitude raises yet another problem in this type of research. Discourse analysts argue that it is time to abandon the notion of consistency at the level of the individual and instead examine the complex and flexible nature of linguistic constructions used by participants, and the consequences of these constructions.

This point can be demonstrated best by examining responses to questions concerning health care for Asian women. A frequent repertoire that emerged here was that of 'cultural differences'. This repertoire is based on the notion that Asian women's choices and practices will be informed by their cultural grouping. In many cases carers expressed uncertainty about being sufficiently informed about cultural differences and discussed the need to be educated about culture to allow them to provide satisfactory care. The extracts below illustrate this 'cultural differences' repertoire.

> *Health visitor 9*: Health visitors need to be well informed about different cultural practices. Then it's possible to go in to a mother and know what to tell her about feeding her baby and what foods she should eat, and educate her effectively. If you don't know anything about Asian food then you can't tell an Asian woman what she should be feeding her child.

> *Health visitor 1*: I'd like some advance warning and try to find out about their religion in relation to diet. If they are vegetarian or not, to know what sort of milk, if they are breastfeeding, although I do know that they (Asian women) prefer to bottle feed milk.

> *Midwife 1*: Asian women don't have any progressive ideas about childbirth. They just lie on their backs and moan. It's not much fun having a woman just lie and whine at you. You know when you first walk in that they'll just want to lie down and get it over with.

These extracts share the perspective that differences based on culture are to be expected. The first extracts produce the argument that once well informed about culture, health carers will be able to provide good care for Asian women. These three extracts make the assumption that all Asian women will behave and act in the same way, because they belong to the same cultural grouping. In the second extract the implication is that the health visitor knows about a woman's feeding preferences simply by knowing her cultural grouping. The assumption in the first extract is that Asian women will eat Asian food, no

246 246

mention is given of finding out what diet an Asian woman chooses for herself and her baby. This might seem a minor point but it can be seen to provide a different discussion of good practice than that provided by 'individualized care'. Here concern for finding out about individual wishes and needs is missing. This extract does *not* refer to establishing a partnership with decisions resting with mothers, but instead sees control as coming from the health carer. The third extract provides an illustration of a negative generalization being made that all Asian women do not have 'progressive ideas' about childbirth. Again, no mention is included of asking Asian mothers about choices about childbirth; the midwife says that she 'knows' what to expect.

Thus, there is a disjunction between the two repertoires of 'individualized care' and 'cultural differences'. More specifically it can be argued that the use of the 'cultural differences' repertoire compromises that of individualized care. Individualized care was so frequently made use of by carers as they discussed good care that it seemed to be almost taken for granted, or common sense. However, the conceptualization is limited when it is not used in discussing good care for *all* women. While being informed about different practices, whether based on culture or religion, to facilitate the health carer's ability to meet individual need, this understanding needs to be integrated with that of individualized care so that all women are first asked about their wishes and choices, and the health carer respects and responds to those choices.

Finally, where the assumption is made that all women who belong to a particular group will adopt the same practices around childbirth and childcare, a gross stereotype comes into play which once again serves to deny women from ethnic minority groups the care which is appropriate to their individual needs and wishes.

CONCLUSION

There are a number of points to be made following this brief examination of health carers' accounts. First, it can be argued that attitude scales provide a blunt instrument for the examination of conceptualizations of health care which serve to obscure rather than reveal the complexity of discussions. Second, the notion that individuals can be placed in discrete categories of positive or negative attitudes would seem to be misconceived. This examination of carers' understandings shows that those same individuals who clearly positively support 'individualized care' also draw on discussions of care which stand in contradiction and undermine ideas of attending to individual needs and choices. Attitude scales are limited in that they examine only one aspect of practice at a time, and cannot allow consideration of the complex inter-relation of ideas.

The rationale behind attitudinal research in this area is to differentiate between health carers with negative attitudes and those with positive attitudes. It had been stated that this will allow for the bias of selection processes so that those individuals with negative attitudes are not appointed for midwifery or health visiting posts (Todman and Jauncey, 1987). This is said to be a more effective solution than opting for retraining programmes.

Discourse analysis suggests an alternative view. Rather than seeing the 'problem' as residing within those individual health carers with 'bad attitudes', discourse analysts direct attention at training structures. If carers do not have discourses made available to them which set out ways in which individualized care can be applied to *all* mothers and which also allow an integration of understanding of cultural differences which does *not* undermine that of individualized care, then their conceptualizations of good care will be limited.

If good care is set up in policy documents as comprising particular practices with a certain relationship set up between carer and client, then it is important to see whether this is the same as that integrated in training programmes and whether health carers draw on this same conceptualization as they discuss their work. These accounts show that given the frequency with which carers drew on 'individualized care', it would seem that this is being communicated to a certain extent. However, the conceptualization is restricted, in that the repertoire was abandoned when discussing care for women from ethnic minority groups. Here a different notion of good care was adopted, which serves to undermine individualized care. What is needed is a rethinking of training programmes so that the various aspects currently thought to characterize good care are fully articulated in varying contexts and in relation to different client groups. Research is then needed to examine whether health carers are making good use of these discourses as they discuss their work.

REFERENCES

Association of Radical Midwives (1986) *The Vision: Proposals for the future of the maternity services*, Association of Radical Midwives, Ormskirk.
Birch, P. (1982) Mothers' decision-making during labour and delivery, unpublished Masters thesis, McGill University, Montreal.
Chapman, C. (1983) The paradox of nursing, *Journal of Advanced Nursing*, **8**, 269–72.
Fishbein, M. and Azjen, I. (1975) *Belief, Attitude, Intention and Behaviour: An introduction to theory and research* Addison-Wesley, Reading, MA.
Gould, D. (1990) Empathy: A review of the literature with suggestions for an alternative research strategy, *Journal of Advanced Nursing*, **15**, 1167–74.
Marshall, H. (1992) Talking about good maternity care in a multicultural context: A discourse analysis of the accounts of midwives and health visitors, in P. Nicolson and J. Ussher (eds.) *The Psychology of Women's Health and Health Care*, Macmillan, London.
Morales-Mann, E.T. (1989) Comparative analysis of the perceptions of patients and nurses about the importance of nursing activities in a postpartum unit, *Journal of Advanced Nursing*, **14**, 478–84.
Potter, J. and Wetherell, M. (1987) *Discourse Analysis and Social Psychology*, Sage, London.
Royal College of Midwives (1987) *The Role and Education of the Future Midwife in the United Kingdom*, Royal College of Midwives, London.
Shields, D. (1978) Nursing care in labour and patient satisfaction: A descriptive study, *Journal of Advanced Nursing*, **3**, no.3, 535–50.
Sparling, S.L. and Jones, S.L. (1977) Setting: A contextual variable associated with empathy, *Journal of Psychiatric and Mental Health Services*, **15**, 9–12.
Todman, J. and Jauncey, L. (1987) Student and qualified midwives' attitudes to aspects of obstetric practice, *Journal of Advanced Nursing*, **12**, 49–55.
United Kingdom Central Council for Nursing, Midwifery and Health Visiting (1986) *Project 2000: A new preparation for practice*, UKCC, London.

The author would like to acknowledge the support of the *ESRC*

17

The case study

Jonathan Smith

I hope that you can gain two things from this chapter: guidance on carrying out your own case studies, and information on the role of the case study in psychology. The first part of the chapter will discuss some of the ways in which a case study can be performed. I will then use my own research on identity change during pregnancy as an illustration. Finally I will address some more general questions to do with the case study; for example, how can it be related to existing knowledge?

THE PLACE OF THE CASE STUDY IN PSYCHOLOGY

A case study can be conducted at a number of levels, for example:

1. The speech therapist might be concerned with the stuttering of one adolescent.
2. The nurse might want to record the relations of medical staff and patients on just one ward.
3. The anthropologist may be interested in the kinship patterns of one remote tribe.

Despite the very different questions and levels of enquiry, these different projects share a methodological position. For the moment at least, they are interested in examining in great detail, for example, this particular piece of behaviour or this particular problem. How this relates to the behaviour of others is either subordinate or not relevant.

Research adopting the case study approach has been

surprisingly neglected in academic psychology. Why? Perhaps the main answer lies in psychology's wish to emulate the natural sciences with what is perceived as being their concern with the universal and general, and the employment of appropriately rigorous statistical measurements. Ironically then a number of philosophers of science point to a much more pluralistic definition of what science is for and how it is done. So as Gordon Allport points out:

> 'Again and again we meet the biased and superficial objection that personal documents are not, and cannot be, scientifically employed because they deal with single cases ... This objection ... is based upon a narrowly conventional view of what scientific method must be. Whatever contributes to a knowledge of human activity is an admissable method to science.'
>
> (Allport, 1951, p. 140)

Graham (1986) gives an accessible introduction to some of this debate, and Harré (1979, Chapter 7) provides a discussion of the technical arguments for the case study level of enquiry.

So the case study clearly has a place in the human and social sciences. What methods are available to the health professional wanting to conduct a case study?

USEFUL METHODS FOR CASE STUDIES

In this section I will introduce and briefly describe a number of methods which can be used in the psychological case study. What these methods share is their ability to look at the individual in his or her own terms without reference to a comparison group. For details of some additional methods, see Allport (1962).

Interviews

The interview obviously gives a great deal of flexibility to the case study researcher. Normally the interview will be unstructured or semi-structured allowing the investigator to follow up particular points of interest as they arise. Generally it is best to tape-record interviews and transcribe them (very time-consuming!) as this allows subsequent detailed analysis of themes.

Personal documents

This includes the analysis of, for example, diaries, autobiographies, clinical notes. The documents may be pre-existing or elicited from the participant during the study. An example from psychology: Allport (1965) analysed a corpus of *Letters from Jenny*, looking for common patterns in the letters in order to construct a picture of her overall personality.

Interviews and personal documents allow for the possibility of either 'quantitative' or 'qualitative' analysis. The former might take the form of frequency counts or statistical content analysis; the latter a more open response to themes emerging in the text. For a useful 'how to' text on interview technique and qualitative analysis, see Taylor and Bogdan (1984). For an introduction to the role of personal documents in research, see Plummer (1983).

Twenty statements test (TST)

The participant is asked to give twenty answers to the question 'Who am I?' (e.g. I am a nurse, I am a woman, I am optimistic) and then various analyses of the responses can be performed, e.g. categorizing them into groups, looking at the order of response. In practice, a single TST would be unlikely to form the basis of a case study. There are a number of possibilities: a number of TSTs could be elicited from the same person over time to look for changes in self-perception or presentation; or the TST could be used alongside other methods to draw a broader canvas of the participant. An example in practice: a physiotherapist might be interested in whether therapy was related to changes in physical, bodily references in the TST. For more on the TST, see Gordon (1968).

Repertory grids

The repertory grid was devised by George Kelly (1963) as a method for tapping the way an individual perceives or constructs her or his personal and social world. It provides individual (idiographic) yet quantitative data.

In a repertory grid exercise, the participant is presented with a set of cards displaying 'elements' representing important 'characters' – aspects of themselves and key others in their life (e.g. self, ideal self, mother) – and is asked to make comparisons between different combinations of these elements. In practice the participant is usually shown three cards at a time and asked to say how two of them are similar and different from the third. The terms the participant uses are described as constructs and Kelly argues that they provide a clue as to how people see themselves and the world in which they live. The important point about the method when carried out this way is that the participant rather than the investigator comes up with his or her own particular terms of comparison. Once constructs have been elicited, various other procedures and analyses can be performed. An example in practice: a doctor might find it helpful to ascertain a patient's personal constructs when deciding the course of treatment most likely to be accepted by the patient. Bannister and Fransella (1986) give an introduction to the use of repertory grids.

Triangulation

Triangulation is a method of drawing on evidence from different sources, and interpreting some in the light of others. This can give a richer, more detailed picture of the person. For example, one can see if themes emerging from interview data are supported, extended or contradicted by constructs obtained from a repertory grid. I used triangulation in a study of pregnancy and identity (Smith, 1990b) which I describe in the next section.

CLARE: A CASE STUDY OF IDENTITY AND THE TRANSITION TO MOTHERHOOD

My main interest in this project was in the way in which a woman's sense of self changed during the transition to motherhood. I wanted to produce a detailed account of each case, trying to do justice to the complexity and multifarious nature of the transition. Here I will talk about how I conducted one case study, and illustrate some of the findings. This summary of the case partly draws on already published material (Smith, 1990a, 1991).

I visited Clare four times at about three, six and nine months

Table 17.1 *Schedule of data collected during Clare's pregnancy*

Visit 1 (3 months)	Visit 2 (6 months)	Visit 3 (9 months)
Interview 1	Interview 2	Interview 3
Diary ———————————————————————→		
Rep Grid 1	Rep Grid 2	Rep Grid 3
TST1		TST2

pregnant and five months after the birth of her first child, and collected several pieces of data at each visit. Because of space limitations, I will only talk about some of the data I collected during the pregnancy here. Table 17.1 shows the schedule for this material.

The interviews were semi-structured. I asked Clare about how she felt the pregnancy was affecting her sense of identity, about her relationships with key others and so on. Between visits she kept a diary of things that occurred to her to do with the topics raised in the interviews.

At the beginning of her pregnancy, Clare was 29 and in full-time employment. She is married to Paul, who is considerably older than her, and who is the father of a child from a previous relationship. The names of the woman and members of her family have been changed to protect confidentiality.

The repertory grids

I need to give some more details of how this part of the study was conducted. I chose elements that I hoped would help elicit the woman's views on how the pregnancy was affecting her sense of identity. The elements were:

1. Me on my own
2. Me at a meal with friends
3. Myself at 12
4. My ideal self
5. Myself as I expect to be in one year's time
6. My mother now
7. My father now
8. My partner
9. Somebody I dislike

The elements were presented to Clare in groups of three, as previously discussed. Eight sets of comparisons produced eight constructs (e.g. resilient, progressive). Clare then rated each construct as it applied to each element (scale 0–10). This then tells us how important she thinks each of the constructs is as a description of each of the key figures. The rating was then repeated at each subsequent visit.

When analysing the grids, I looked at the relationship between constructs, and between elements, within a grid and over time. Thus we can see, for example, how close a woman feels to her ideal self by looking at the correlation of the scores given for those two elements on a grid. We can also see how that correlation changes over time to see whether a woman feels more, or less, like her ideal self through the transition to motherhood. Thus using repertory grids one can gain a vast amount of information about one person, in her own terms, without reference to other participants or pre-existing statistical norms.

I wanted to present this information graphically to the individual woman. Therefore I drew a diagram (Figure 17.1) which has lines connecting those constructs which are significantly correlated on a particular grid. By plotting the relationships for all the grids for one woman on the same sheet, we can see how these construct relations change through time. I then repeated this exercise for the elements. I hope the reader is also able to see the pattern emerging in the diagram, the content of which will be discussed below.

I have selected two themes which illustrate the value of triangulation, where one can see the same idea being played out in different sources:

1. Pregnancy as psychological preparation for mothering.
2. Increasing involvement with key others, culminating in the development of a relational self: a stronger sense of self as informed by engagement with important others.

Pregnancy as psychological preparation for mothering

Clare seems to use her pregnancy as a time for psychological preparation for childbirth and becoming a mother. She speaks at three months pregnant of the need to prepare herself 'for

three months pregnant

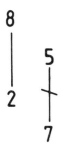

six months pregnant

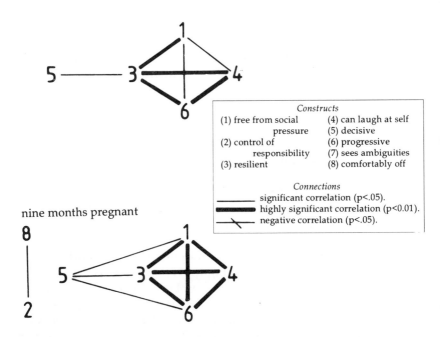

Constructs

(1) free from social pressure
(2) control of responsibility
(3) resilient
(4) can laugh at self
(5) decisive
(6) progressive
(7) sees ambiguities
(8) comfortably off

Connections

―――― significant correlation (p<.05).
▬▬▬ highly significant correlation (p<0.01).
―✗― negative correlation (p<.05).

nine months pregnant

Figure 17.1 Changing pattern of construct correlations over time. Lines connect constructs which are correlated.

what lies ahead', a movement away from external concerns with work, because:

'there is a need to, not withdraw within yourself, but just to prepare, and to make ready and to make sure that you are whole.'

By six months we can see how confidence gained from a period of self-containment seems to be helping Clare in her preparation for becoming a mother:

'I'm beginning to feel my bulk though (laughs) and slowing down and generally very level ... stately as a galleon ... I'm not getting flapped about things or whatever, you just sort of sail on ... I've developed more confidence, not in an overt self-confident way. I'm just ... more self contained.'

Perhaps physical weight helps prepare for psychological weight and depth.

At nine months pregnant, Clare presents herself as more questioning, uncertain and impatient:

'This emergence of a new life is very near and impending now, whereas whenever it was back in June, was a sort of floating ... Having to come out of that, I suppose it's a sort of protection which I'm having to break free of now in order to move on to the next stage ... The ground is much more uncertain than it was three months ago. You reach out for it but you wonder and you can't wait for it.'

Generally, then, Clare's focus is moving outwards again. She is emerging from containment, and the coming birth seems to be the main catalyst to this change. It would appear that the self-containing acted as a protection which will help strengthen Clare for the next stage but which now needs to be thrown off as Clare is looking uncertainly, and with some trepidation, to the immediate future.

The theme of 'containment' gains some support from the repertory grid data – see Figure 17.1. Through the pregnancy there is an increase in the number of connections between constructs. What this means is that constructs implicate each other: if Clare sees a person as 'resilient' she also sees her or him as 'progressive' and so on. Thus there is a narrowing or focusing of terms, coincident with Clare's preparatory self-containing.

In terms of content, the term which comes to mind to describe the cluster of constructs at six months pregnant is 'being together'; that is, Clare views people in terms of how 'together' they are, this being made up of the constructs: free from social pressures (C1), resilient (C3), can laugh at self (C4), and progressive (C6). By nine months pregnant 'decisive' (C5) joins this cluster. Again there is a connection with the qualitative material – there is obviously a close correspondence between being 'contained' and being 'together'.

Thus during the pregnancy this notion tightens its grip but its definition gains a harder edge with the inclusion of 'resilience' and then 'decisiveness', this change corresponding to the need to steel herself for the birth, discussed in the interview material.

The development of the relational self

There is a growing sense of psychological relationship with key others during the pregnancy. During the interviews and diaries we see Clare talking more, explicitly or implicitly, about involvement with key others: partner, mother, sister. Thus, for example, at three months Clare speaks of how the pregnancy is likely to draw her mother and her closer:

'I will have entered the elite – no, not the elite, er – the band of women, if you see what I mean. Motherhood is very important to her and I think the fact that I will be sharing that experience will make a difference to her.

It's almost as if actually having a child makes the relationship much more equal ... I think there'll be more a feeling of assuredness ... in my relationship, as an adult, with my mother.'

At six months we see Clare describing, in her diary, how she is catching up with her husband:

'I managed to get Paul to go to one of the parentcraft sessions run at the health centre ... Somehow I wanted the reassurance of public acknowledgement that we're going through this together, it's as if sometimes I feel like I'm running to catch up with him on the experience stakes – pretty inevitable really when you consider the circumstances!'

What emerges is a sense of increasing psychological connections with these key others and a story of her catching up with them, as she moves to the parent status they've already achieved.

Interestingly this experiential sharing is also translated into psychological similarity; that is, Clare sees herself as becoming more similar to her mother and partner. This is captured in the repertory grid data.

three months pregnant

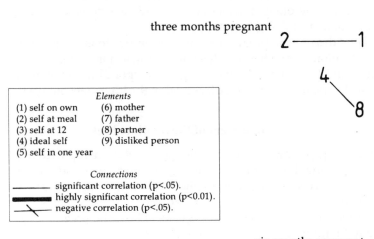

Elements

(1) self on own   (6) mother
(2) self at meal   (7) father
(3) self at 12   (8) partner
(4) ideal self   (9) disliked person
(5) self in one year

Connections

———— significant correlation (p<.05).
▬▬▬ highly significant correlation (p<0.01).
——✕— negative correlation (p<.05).

six months pregnant

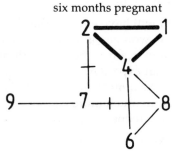

nine months pregnant

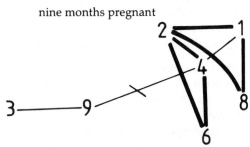

Figure 17.2 Changing pattern of element correlations over time. Lines connect elements which are correlated.

Overall, the element intercorrelation pattern (Figure 17.2) shows a similar trend to that for the constructs; that is, a tightening of connections over time. A connection between two elements means that Clare perceives them as being similar psychologically.

The most striking story in Figure 17.2 is the growing connections of mother and partner with self. Her partner's links at six months pregnant are to mother (element E6), father (E7) and ideal self (E4). At nine months these are replaced by highly significant connections with self alone (E1) and self with friends (E2). Thus it would appear that her partner is now described in terms of the immediate self rather than a more distant parental or ideal figure. He is being 'drawn in' (Clare's words) to play a central part in Clare's personal construct world. A similar movement happens to 'mother'.

Thus Clare would seem to have 'caught up' relationally, experientially and psychologically: the relationships are closer, she shares more with Paul and her mother, and they are now more like her psychologically.

These two themes hint at the complex process of pregnancy. On the one hand we see a need to look inwards away from the public world, as preparation for mothering. On the other hand we see increased engagement with family members. Thus it may be for Clare that she needed to turn away from the public world of work, to have a period of self-containment, but that that period of containment also required, or led to, closer contact with those most important to her.

The net effect of these processes is, at nine months, some recognition of changing identity, the greater importance to her sense of self of the relationships she is engaged in:

'I'm me but I'm one of two and I'm also one of three ... and the emphasis is always changing ... Sometimes you feel as though me is being lost or submerged ... On the whole me is intact but I don't think I want to be me on my own entirely for ever more anyway, I mean, how do you explain it? An irrevocable decision, the steps have been made that mean that my other identities, if you like, as a mother and as a partner make up that essential me now.'

The passage makes a strong statement about a shift in Clare's perception of her identity, her roles as mother and partner

Table 17.2 *Twenty Statements Test responses*

Visit 1: three months pregnant

A Conscientious
   Methodical
   Precise   *Key*
   Have a long fuse   A Attribute
   Over-analytical   B State
   Indecisive   C Physical
   Late   D Existential
   Infuriating   E Group identity
   Lazy   F Relational
   Loving
   Loyal

B Happy
   Lucky
   Calm
   Pregnant

C Blonde
   Well-built
   Short-sighted

D Me

E Female

Visit 3: nine months pregnant

B Happy
   Incredible
   Looking forward
   Intrigued
   Apprehensive
   Wondering what is going to happen
   Wondering
   Wanting to get on with it
   Torn in different directions – sometimes
   More simple minded most of the time
   Mixed up
   Emotional

C Feeling very large
   Feeling very slow
   Lumbering

F A mother
   A partner
   One of two twice
   One of three

Table 17.3 *Twenty Statements Test – results of informal categorization*

		3m	9m
A	Attribute	11	-
B	State	4	13
C	Physical	3	3
D	Existential	1	-
E	Group identity	1	-
F	Social relations	-	4

becoming more central to her sense of self. Perhaps part of moving on and away from self-containment is the growing recognition of the importance of one's role in relation to others. That this is not an easy process is suggested by the ambivalence in Clare's reaction.

Catching up with her partner and her own mother has partly facilitated recognition of self as mother. Public acknowledgment of the new status of family which comes from, for example, joint attendance at the antenatal class further enhances the new emphasis on relational roles.

Twenty Statements Test

What light do the TSTs shed on the picture? Table 17.2 shows the responses, categorized according to my informal classification scheme, and Table 17.3 the results of this categorization.

Two confirmations come from the TSTs. Firstly we can see the concern with the immediate future arising at nine months pregnant; many responses express the mixed feelings about the coming birth (e.g. apprehensive, wanting to get on with it). Secondly we can see some confirmation of the importance of the relational self at nine months, in the inclusion of four relational identity statements where there were none at three months pregnant.

Overall, the TSTs add their own particular dimension in emphasizing the extent of the shifting nature of Clare's self-perception in response to pregnancy. At three months pregnant most of Clare's responses are general trait or attribute statements (e.g. methodical, precise). She is telling us about her long-standing individual personality characteristics. There is only one statement about pregnancy – 'pregnant'. The responses at nine months pregnant are very different. There is a reversal from trait to state descriptions. Some of these are clearly about pregnancy (e.g. wanting to get on with it) and all of the others could also be interpreted as being about the pregnancy (e.g. mixed up). The three physical descriptions are all to do with pregnancy (e.g. lumbering).

Summary

The case material portrays Clare's pregnancy as a complex developmental phase, and as psychological preparation for mothering. This preparation takes the form of a shift from the public world of, for example, work to the more intimate world of self and important others. This change can be seen reflected in the different data sources. Clare talks of the need to have time for self-containment before the rupture of childbirth; this is mirrored by the emergence of 'being together' as a key system in her personal construct data.

Towards the end of pregnancy, Clare emerges from containment to face the looming birth. Her interview reflects some mixed feelings including trepidation; the personal construct system takes on a harder edge; the TSTs are dominated by concerns around the birth.

The development of the relational self, an identity facilitated by and grounded in relations with key others, also emerges from all data sources, appearing in how Clare talks and writes about the growing importance of her relations with key others, in the convergences in the repertory grid data, and in the new inclusion of role statements in her TST at nine months pregnant.

WHAT CAN YOU DO WITH A CASE STUDY?

Firstly, we should remember that the case study is important in its own right. I would like to stress that, because of psychology's neglect of enquiries at this level, there is the need for detailed studies of individuals in their own terms, attempting to capture their complexity, and possibly ambiguity, through intensive in-depth studies. Clare's study can actually stand alone as a testament to the complex inter-relationship between becoming a mother and one's sense of identity.

One can go beyond the case itself, however. The case study can be used to interrogate existing theory. For example, a single case study might be used to demonstrate that the existing theory is too simple and suggest how it might be revised in the light of this more detailed data.

One can also conduct a number of case studies and begin to use the emerging data base as a powerful theoretical tool. This body of case studies can be used either to test existing theory or to begin to formulate new theory. Methodologically, the argument is that a theory which emerges from the detailed examination of individual cases in their own terms, that is, with as little preconceived categorization as possible, is more likely to do justice to the complexity of the group one is interested in.

In my project on pregnancy I used a small number of case studies, each as detailed as Clare's, to both these ends. For example, I suggested that the trend I found during pregnancy of a turn both to self and also to key others altered the notion of pregnancy as a time of introspection found in the existing literature. The notion of a relational self, of the identity of self intimately bound up with important others, emerged from the detailed analysis of patterns existing in each of the case studies.

Examples in practice: (1) One might find that a case study conducted with a stroke patient begins to raise questions about the guiding principles of occupational therapy. Suggested changes in the existing theory can be made to incorporate the conflicting evidence. (2) Physiotherapy with a new group of patients might lead one to see patterns emerging for the group, and the requirement for the creation of new theory in terms of this particular client group. For more on the role of the case study in research, see Platt (1988); on grounding theory in intensive data analysis, see Strauss (1987).

RESEARCH AS THERAPY, THERAPY AS RESEARCH

Interestingly and perhaps not surprisingly, given the intensity of the exercise, Clare speaks of some therapeutic gain from taking part in the project:

'In a way I am glad that I have done this because it's stripping away those strategies, seeing how I operate, or how I have operated... I will go away and think about it, and I might employ those same strategies again to think, or I may use it to modify how I operate.'

Thus one might say that the amount of self-reflection demanded of a participant, over an extended period, in this sort of project can in itself be therapeutic. Similarly I would like to turn that statement on its head. I would suggest that therapists and other practitioners in the caring professions can be said to be conducting case studies with their clients: the intensive examination of a person, or a particular issue of that person, in their own terms. The reason I am making this point is that too often research and practice are seen as entirely different enterprises, whereas I would suggest that this need not be the case. The presentation of a detailed set of case studies (case notes more formally written up) may provide at least as valid a basis for psychological theorizing as the results obtained from an orthodox psychological inventory distributed by the 'researcher' to a large population. Similarly, single case studies can be seen as providing their own contribution to knowledge, and written up for publication. For a recent example in psychology, see Watts' (1990) clinical case study. I would encourage all practitioners to see the potential for bridging the gap between research and practice in this way.

Note

The author's research reported in this chapter was conducted with the support of a postgraduate studentship from the Economic and Social Research Council. Figures 17.1 and 17.2 are modified versions of figures first appearing in Smith (1990a).

REFERENCES

Allport, G.W. (1951) *The Use Of Personal Documents In Psychological Science*, Social Science Research Council, (Bulletin No. 49), New York.

Allport, G.W. (1962) The general and the unique in psychological science, *Journal of Personality*, **30**, 405–22.

Allport, G.W. (1965) *Letters from Jenny*, Harcourt, New York.

References 265

Bannister, D. and Fransella, F. (1986) *Inquiring Man: The psychology of personal constructs*, 3rd edn, Croom Helm, London.

Gordon, C. (1968) Self-conceptions: Configurations of content, in C. Gordon and K.J. Gergen (eds.) *The Self in Social Interaction*, Wiley, New York.

Graham, H. (1986) *The Human Face of Psychology*, Open University Press, Milton Keynes.

Harré, R. (1979) *Social Being*, Blackwell, Oxford.

Kelly, G.A. (1963) *A Theory of Personality: The psychology of personal constructs*, Norton, New York.

Platt, J. (1988) What can case studies do? in R.G. Burgess (ed.) *Studies in Qualitative Methodology: A research annual: Conducting qualitative research, Vol 1*, JAI Press, Greenwich, Connecticut.

Plummer, K. (1983) *Documents of Life: An introduction to the problems and literature of humanistic method*, Allen and Unwin, London.

Smith, J.A. (1990a) Transforming identities: A repertory grid case-study of the transition to motherhood, *British Journal of Medical Psychology*, **63**, 239–53.

Smith, J.A. (1990b) Self-construction: Longitudinal studies in the psychology of personal identity and life transitions, unpublished D. Phil thesis, University of Oxford.

Smith, J.A. (1991) Conceiving selves: A case study of changing identities during the transition to motherhood, *Journal of Language and Social Psychology*, **10**, 225–43.

Strauss, A. (1987) *Qualitative Analysis for Social Scientists*, Cambridge University Press, Cambridge.

Taylor, S. and Bogdan, R. (1984) *Introduction to Qualitative Research Methods*, 2nd edn, Wiley, New York.

Watts, F. (1990) Aversion to body hair: A case study in the integration of behavioural and interpretative methods, *British Journal of Medical Psychology*, **63**, 335–40.

Author index

Subject index